Functionality and Efficient Services Delivery in Nigerian Hospitals

Edited by

Inyang Ukot
RST Clinics Ltd.
Federal Housing Estate
Uyo, Akwa Ibom State, Nigeria

Functionality and Efficient Services Delivery in Nigerian Hospitals

Editor: Inyang Ukot

ISBN (Online): 979-8-89881-204-1

ISBN (Print): 979-8-89881-205-8

ISBN (Paperback): 979-8-89881-206-5

Published by Bentham Science Publishers Pte. Ltd. Singapore, in collaboration with Eureka Conferences, USA.

First published in 2026.

Bentham Science Publishers Pte. Ltd.
No. 9 Raffles Place
Office No. 26-01
Singapore 048619
Singapore
Email: subscriptions@benthamscience.net

BENTHAM SCIENCE

CONTENTS

FOREWORD

Dr. Inyang Ukot graduated from the College of Medicine of the University of Lagos, Nigeria, with a Bachelor of Medicine and Bachelor of Surgery (MB, BS) in 1981. He completed a residency in Family Medicine and is a Fellow in Family Medicine of the National Postgraduate Medical College of Nigeria (1991) and the West African College of Physicians (1995). He obtained the postgraduate Diploma in Occupational Medicine from the Royal College of Physicians of London in 2005. He was the coordinator of training in Family Medicine at the National Postgraduate Medical College of Nigeria between 1995 and 1999.

Dr. Inyang Ukot has extensive experience as a family medicine specialist and first contact specialist in the health care system, a career spanning about 40 years in Nigeria. This extensive experience and exposure covered health care systems in the North, South, East and West of Nigeria, a highly populated developing nation in Sub-Saharan Africa. In the first year of his career, Inyang worked in Eku Baptist Hospital, located in a rural area in the South-South part of Nigeria; and during his year of compulsory service (NYSC) in Nigeria, he worked in a State government secondary care medical facility in Birnin-Gwari in the North-Central part of Nigeria. During his residency in Family Medicine, he had a stint in a Presbyterian Church hospital in the South-South part of Nigeria, NKST Church hospital and two Catholic Church hospitals in Benue State (North-Central part of Nigeria). Dr Inyang Ukot was the first family physician to head the General Outpatients' Department of the University of Port Harcourt Teaching Hospital in the capital city of the oil-producing Rivers State in the early '90s. In the mid-nineties, he was one of the two specialists who led the medical services department of United Bank for Africa (UBA) in UBA House, Lagos Island, Lagos State. He worked in two busy, high-profile private hospitals in Ikeja, Lagos State, in the southwest of Nigeria between 1992 and 1996, and between 1998 and 2006, he was a staff physician for ExxonMobil in Nigeria.

Dr. Ukot's vast work experience covers primary, secondary, and tertiary health care and hospitals. He has worked in hospitals in rural areas, semi-urban areas, and cities in Nigeria for over 40 years. He is well aware of the details of the structure and function/malfunction of the health care system and hospitals in Nigeria. The contents of this multi-author book, with chapters authored by well-chosen specialists are a valuable resource for current and prospective foreign and local investors in healthcare, proprietors, professionals, policymakers, regulators of medical training and practice, and patients in any setting in any developing country. He commenced the writing of his first book in medicine one year after completing his postgraduate training in Family Medicine, a writing career with publishing dates in 1996 and 2023. Many medical students have benefited from his MCQ book.

Inyang is, therefore, well experienced in writing **Functionality and Efficient Services Delivery in Nigerian Hospitals**, a book I recommend to all stakeholders in the Nigerian healthcare system and other sub-Saharan countries.

Emmanuel Monjok
Primary care and Community Medicine
University of Calabar and University of Calabar Teaching hospital
Calabar, Nigeria

PREFACE

Functionality and Efficient Services Delivery in Nigerian Hospitals arose from the author's observations during his over-forty-years medical practice, which covers the north, south, east, and west of Nigeria. The summary of the observations is that while there have been remarkable improvements and advancement in almost every segment of their societies, the advancement in medical facilities and medical services in Nigeria and many developing countries has lagged significantly – and the degree of dropping back in comparison with the status in the advanced countries seems that there is no hope of catching up unless Nigeria and similar countries make a definite and deliberate attempt at addressing this sore thumb. Dr. Ukot and his team believe that this situation can be resolved and that is why they joined hands to pen this book in a way that is easy to read and understand its contents and implement the suggestions it proffers; this is because of its deliberate a small volume that makes this work "friendly" enough for every reader to read in its entirety. This book is a combination of "saying it as it is" and "crying and hoping to be heard" while keeping in mind the beneficiaries of the goings on in our hospitals – the patients and the employees.

The title of this book, Functionality and Efficient Services Delivery in Nigerian Hospitals, is specific and the book limits itself to that. This book intends to cover, and therefore only deals with, the area of the goings-on in medical facilities and the various influences or factors that determine the structure, function, and clientele of hospitals in developing countries using Nigeria as the prototype.

In this book, the word "Hospital" encompasses facilities as small as health posts and health centers and large ones like tertiary hospitals, of which teaching hospitals are good examples. It is difficult to write on even the teaching hospitals in Nigeria as they belong to different "generations" in terms of age, equipment profile, staff strength, land and facility sizes, level and structure of personnel, administrative focus and style, and the peculiarities and diversity of the patients and third parties that patronize the hospitals. It was, consequently, very difficult to choose the four hospitals whose stories are told in this book – two of them are teaching hospitals and the other two are private hospitals. Of the two teaching hospitals, one is a Federal government-owned hospital, while the other is owned and run by a Christian Mission. With reference to the private hospitals, one is a medium-sized hospital, while the other is a small hospital. Each of them has an interesting story and they provide us with examples of making things work in similar existing or future hospitals. It was not difficult to choose some of the authors because they readily saw the need for the project when they were approached; it was difficult to eventually obtain consent to write from others as many declined due to time constraints in writing to meet deadlines. The completed work reflects the original intention and it is hoped that this work will be of assistance to every reader as it has a message for everyone.

Inyang Ukot
RST Clinics Ltd.
Federal Housing Estate
Uyo, Akwa Ibom State, Nigeria

ACKNOWLEDGMENTS

When I approached the co-authors of this book, I was not certain that they would buy the idea considering the fact that the book is neither a novel nor a medical textbook; moreover, some of them are specialists in areas that are outside medicine. To my surprise, and their credit, they all agreed to contribute to this peculiar book. I am grateful to them for carving out time out of their busy schedules to enrich this work. The book has turned out to be a well-woven material that will benefit healthcare services delivery by managers/operators and the various professionals in medical facilities in Nigeria.

Being the Ultimate, I acknowledge God for providing the idea, good health and fortitude that enabled me not only to conceive this work but also to start the writing, coordination and organization of chapter contributions and eventual production of this book – overcoming the numerous challenges in between.

DEDICATION

To our immediate family members who have supported us in our professional and personal endeavors, our colleagues with whom we have grown over the years, our mentees who have accepted and benefited from the impartations from us, and our numerous patients to whom we have committed our best although we may not have saved all.

INTRODUCTION

Abstract: Hospitals are a key component of the system for health care delivery in any country. In Nigeria and other developing parts of the world, it is not different. Hospitals may be seen as the last part of a chain or cascade of institutions that are established to provide appropriate services for the well and the ill. "The well" is mentioned before "the ill" because until the populace, healthcare system designers, and operators remember or factor in this fact, we shall continue to be inundated with people with illness rather than prevent illness and promote health. When there is a combination of illness prevention and health promotion, service providers, hospital facilities, equipment, and consumables do not get overstretched.

The starting point in the healthcare delivery system appears to be imprecise. This author thinks that it could be the point of entry into medical schools and other schools that prepare and produce the wide variety of professionals we find in hospitals – and this variety is ever-increasing in number and sub-specialization. The starting point could predate entry into the training institutions and could be taken as the ideas, plans, and actions of various policy makers.

The World Health Organization (WHO), in its Overview on Hospitals, documented that "Hospitals matter to people and often mark central points in their lives. They also matter to health systems by being instrumental in care coordination and integration. They often provide a setting for education of doctors, nurses and other health-care professionals and are a critical base for clinical research."[1] This book chapter, although written in the form of a story, addresses, in generality, the value of the contributions of hospitals to healthcare delivery systems, to the personnel in hospitals, to the clients who patronize hospitals (patients), and to research.

There are several ways to describe or classify hospitals. The following summarizes the classes of hospitals: "Hospitals may be classified by type of service, ownership, size by number of beds, and length of stay" [2].

The European Observatory's work on health care delivery describes health care delivery thus: "Health care delivery forms the most visible function of the health system, both to patients and the general public. It concentrates on patient flows as well as the organization and delivery of all services dealing with the diagnosis and treatment of disease or the promotion, maintenance and restoration of health. It covers the principal areas of service provision such as public health, primary care, specialized care (often divided into secondary and tertiary care), urgent and emergency care, pharmaceutical care, rehabilitation/intermediate care, long-term care, services for informal carers, palliative care, mental health care and dental care" [3].

The approach adopted for this chapter is because every type of hospital is important and the author considers the smallest and the most basic set of hospitals the "foundation" of the system of health care delivery in any part of the world. The foundation of any building determines in incredibly significant terms the viability and safety of that structure, irrespective of how fanciful or attractive it is. The chapter covers hospitals of diverse types and levels, their locations, their operators, and their clients. It concentrates on what happens and should happen in such medical facilities.

Hospitals should not just work, but their various practitioners must cultivate and maintain a culture of continuous improvement. What and who determines that hospitals are functional and rendering efficient services? It is the quality of service delivery that determines that hospitals work, and it is the beneficiaries of the services who can rightly determine that hospitals work. There is no need for the system designers, operators, and monitors to independently conclude that their system works without getting concurring input from the beneficiaries or users of the services and facilities in hospitals.

Keywords: Client services, Design and utilities, Distribution, Federal ministry of health and social welfare, Health insurance schemes, Healthcare personnel, Healthcare sector, Hospitals, Large hospitals, Location, Medium-sized hospitals, Ministries of health, Nigerians, Professional bodies, Public perception, Regulatory bodies, Small hospitals, Training, Work relationships.

HOSPITALS

In Nigeria and other developing countries, there is a diversity of hospitals and they are briefly described.

Types – In terms of diversity, there are health posts, health clinics, maternity homes, health centers, comprehensive health centers, cottage hospitals, general hospitals, specialist hospitals, federal medical centers, and university teaching hospitals. This list may not be comprehensive but suffice it to say that their categorization can be Primary healthcare facilities, Secondary healthcare facilities, and Tertiary healthcare facilities.

Design and Utilities – Facilities management is discussed in detail in Chapter 4. However, before the management of a hospital's physical structure, furniture, furnishing, and equipment, the building must be put up. Ideally, medical facilities should be designed as hospitals and constructed to meet the purpose. This means that detailed consideration should be given to the size of the hospital, projected population it would serve, types, sizes and number of floors of the building(s), and parking space. Various sections of the hospital must be planned to make sense in terms of relationships – the location of the mortuary must certainly not be in proximity to the kitchen or out-patients' department; there should be a natural relationship between the various out-patients' departments just as a similar relationship should be established between the maternity ward, labor ward, and the operating room/theater that serves that wing of the hospital. Such "natural" relationships should be seen in every large hospital and, therefore, be established at the design stage. Minute details must be paid to the walls, roofing, floors, doors, windows, ventilation, lighting, water supply, drainage, signage, ease of access and movement, refuse and sewage disposal, and other considerations. Safety and security considerations must be built into the structure just as provision should be made for expansion if the need arises in the future. Since everything must be factored in and designed to meet the standards of a hospital, it is certainly not good to hurriedly put up a hospital building or building complex; neither is it good practice to use "converted" buildings as hospitals or clinics. It is because of such conversion that a number of hospitals do not have patients' drop-off zones with ramps or ease of use of wheelchairs and trolleys. Some large and busy hospitals do not even have dedicated entry and exit points for in-house and external ambulances to bring in patients and depart with ease. A well-conceived and satisfactorily-constructed hospital facility will have enough space within and outside to meet the needs of its patients, personnel, and third-party service providers. Green areas should be incorporated into the plan of hospitals.

A hospital must have a continuous water supply even if it does not have a continuous electricity supply – having both is ideal, and all developing countries should strive to make these available for their hospitals. In countries where health is taken as a priority indeed, continuous electric power and water supply are sine-qua-non.

Effective maintenance must be built into every hospital or there will be a predictably rapid deterioration of the facility.

Distribution and location – Using Nigeria as not only an example but also a reference, in terms of number, a cursory observation is that where most people reside is sometimes where there are the least number of functional hospitals. This statement sounds incredible at face value when one considers that University Teaching Hospitals located in either State capitals or major cities attend to a lot of patients on a daily basis. If a pregnant woman in a remote part of a state is in obstructed labor and cannot get attention in any nearby hospital and eventually has Cesarean section or instrumental delivery of a stillborn (or both mother and baby die), will the immediate family members count the clinics, medical centers, or general hospitals that they bypassed to get to the nearest Teaching Hospital to receive belated service as hospitals? They ordinarily should not.

For hospitals in Nigeria to demonstrate functionality, deliver efficient services to their clients, and exhibit continuous improvement they may not be evenly distributed but must be well distributed (appropriately distributed) in the entire country. The distribution should be based not only on population but also on proximity to current and prospective end-users in terms of time and space. It is counter-intuitive and improper to site a "big hospital" in a small community like a village just because of political considerations; this could be because the State governor, a senator, or some other politically relevant individual is from that community. Locating a medical facility such that it is isolated from the nearest referral medical facility could be counter-productive. Good intentions aside, that facility is subject to failure if utilities and facilities like public electricity, water, reliable telecommunication, roads, vehicular traffic, fuel stations, and rail systems are not available to readily link their patients who need a referral from the referring center to a referral center.

It defeats the purpose of a hospital for relevant authorities to approve a clinic or hospital to be sited within a shopping complex or business plaza just because such places receive and serve many people daily. It will not serve the intended purpose if a hospital is situated in a congested area such that the hospital does not have adequate car parking grounds for staff and patients. It is also not fair or appropriate to allow hospitals to be sited close to a flood-prone area, landfill, refuse dump site, abattoir, bus station, quarry, or erosion site.

Small hospitals – Small hospitals need not have all the features of large hospitals. They must be designed and equipped to render the services they intended to and are approved to provide and stick to them – or expand appropriately to add other services. One problem in many developing countries, including Nigeria, is that there are not enough small hospitals. Small hospitals may be private clinics/hospitals, or they may be government-owned medical facilities. Ideally, small hospitals should be dotted around every part of a country; each of these small hospitals should be able to meet the needs of the residents in the communities where they are located. A small hospital may actually render primary health services while another small hospital can devote itself to providing high-profile, sub-specialty services; the former fits into rural and semi-urban areas while the latter is ideal for urban centers like large cities, State capitals and nations' capitals. Unfortunately, many small private hospitals are set up with the intention to provide every service – and have every facility. This means that such small hospitals do not see themselves as adequate without having the full diagnostic set-up in terms of the laboratory, radiology, ultrasonography, and operative capability, among other contraptions and services. This author believes that this needs not be. It could simply be because of this type of mindset that prospective investors are not encouraged to set up diagnostic centers within the reach of, say, ten or fifteen small private or government hospitals. If this challenge were not the case, standalone diagnostic centers would be able to run profitably while the small hospitals would not stretch themselves thin and lean, carrying a load beyond their professional, financial, and administrative capacity. The diagnostic centers could give the small hospitals that patronize them discounts based on the level of patronage, to the effect that both parties would benefit financially and professionally. Investors in small hospitals, if they followed this format of operation, would be able to start functional professional medical facilities that render good services with a reasonable budget. Coupled with the assurance of a reasonable and functional referral system they would save the lives of patients with emergency cases as such patients would be stabilized prior to referral. I believe and would recommend that, though these hospitals are private, State and Federal governments should provide such operators a reasonable incentive to site small hospitals in the periphery – rural and remote parts of all the states in the country. This recommendation is based on the stark reality that the cost of running an efficient hospital in a rural area is much higher than in the urban centers where electricity, water, roads, means of transportation and communication are available, even if they are "epileptic." A good distribution of and support system for such hospitals would provide a healthcare service network that would work and save lives; we are witnesses that lives are currently lost unnecessarily before patients arrive at the nearest large hospitals that, in reality, are frequently distant.

Medium-sized hospitals – In-between small hospitals and large hospitals, discussed below, are medium-sized hospitals. In Nigeria, they could be private, company, or government hospitals. Their characteristics tend to be a mix of what is applicable in small and large hospitals. These hospitals are important in Nigeria.

Large hospitals – Large hospitals are being overwhelmed with patients that are supposed to be attended to at the lower strata of the healthcare delivery system; when this situation continues, these hospitals do not function optimally and the structural facilities and equipment are over-used, under-maintained, and rapidly run down. In terms of the buildings, it smacks of poor planning to have hospitals that are on four, five floors, and more and do not have lifts (elevators) – or, when existent, are unreliable or non-functional. When the external and internal walls of any large hospital, particularly government-owned hospitals, look old and dilapidated, it is discouraging to patients, their relatives, visitors, and hospital employees. Such a decrepit outlook of hospitals is not right, even if top-notch services are rendered within. A sad feature of the grounds of many of our large hospitals is their being dotted with uncompleted building projects. In developing countries, uncompleted projects are not only an eyesore but also venues for unwholesome practices, including criminal acts. Security personnel in many of our public hospitals have enough work without the unnecessary addition of keeping an eye on these structures. Sometimes, it takes close to seven years before these projects get to completion – and some give the semblance of abandonment. Many people know of the "hospital smell" of certain hospitals – it is an unwelcome and, sometimes, foreboding smell for many patients, and the odor need not be as it can be prevented or eliminated if proper attention is given to good housekeeping as part of continuous care of the facilities.

Healthcare personnel –Background – The background of every personnel in a medical facility has an impact on the functional or sub-optimal functioning state of such facilities. This is because the output by these core professionals and support staff depends strongly on the mindset of the young people who were trained and eventually found themselves with a career in the healthcare delivery system. Some of us became who we are in this system because we admired one person or the other; had absolutely no idea how the system works, had a good idea of the expectations of the system, or felt constrained to join and stay in the system because we felt we could change the status quo – *i.e.* for people whose significant other like a parent, sibling, *etc.* did not receive what was expected to be the best from a hospital; scored good-to-excellent grades in the high school (secondary school) that qualified us to pick and eventually join any field of our choice in the healthcare sector, *etc.* Most of these reasons do not hold water by the time core hospital personnel start work and meet the unfortunate "realities" on the ground.

Healthcare personnel – Training vis-à-vis work relationships – Before a cleaner, security personnel, medical records officer, laboratory scientist, pharmacist, radiographer, nurse, administrative and management staff, or doctor starts work in any medical facility personnel would have obtained requisite education from various training centers. These training institutions may be at the secondary school (high school) level or university level – or their equivalent. Many of the higher cadre of personnel also have post-graduate academic and/or professional qualifications and have various professional bodies they belong to. It is well-known that the previous sentence holds true for some personnel in the course of service, and not necessarily prior to their being employed to work in hospitals. In spite of the various qualifications, how many of these workers have been specifically trained to work in a hospital setting – having teamwork, understanding of patients and patients' relatives, *etc.* in their training curriculum? The training is usually focused on proficiency that is limited to the respective fields, with a concentration on technical issues. With regard to teamwork, consideration should be given to the fact that the entire hospital workforce must function as a cohesive team; this means that each department and each unit must also work as a team. Is it possible or easy to work as a team when each person has not been trained or received orientation to that effect? Lip service should not be given to this critical issue or allow the fact to be taken for granted. The cardinal role of team work has to be inculcated into the workforce before their joining hospital service or ensured at the earliest stage of every employee's career.

If heads of medical establishments, like chief medical directors, medical directors, and medical superintendents do not see their doctors as colleagues, or all other cadres of employees as key members of their working team, how will a strong chain be formed and maintained? If cleaners, security and janitorial staff or the core clinical personnel have not been trained to see themselves as part-and-parcel of a cohesive functional system, with each employee providing essential services, no hospital can function well consistently. Everybody is important and while some people can do others' work, they will not have the time to do so in the continual absence, inefficiency, or malfunctioning of the others. A doctor, nurse, or pharmacist can certainly do the work of a cleaner (and not *vice-versa*) but they cannot do and continue doing cleaners' work if most of the cleaners are sacked and not replaced or if a cleaner is the only one for the entire clinic, hospital unit, or hospital department. Top management staff, their assistants, heads of department, or supervisors must not harass their subordinates verbally, physically, or emotionally and expect to continue receiving respect, cooperation, and proficiency from them. The team will not function optimally, be it the entire hospital, a department, or unit – and clients will suffer, being on the receiving end of such a dysfunctional state.

Healthcare personnel* – *Client services – One area that separates good medical facilities from the not-so-good ones is client services. Client services is a crux in the life of a medical facility; a hospital must take and treat it as the heart of its practice and business. It is so fundamental that a hospital that pays scant attention to this pivot of medical services would find itself not growing or dropping in rating among its clients. According to the article "Hospital Customer Service: A patient-centered care," "Patient service is key in healthcare in any medical facility. A good patient experience can greatly improve his quality of life, which is the cornerstone of the hospital's success. Accordingly, enhancing the patient's quality of life and focusing on how to improve the medical service provided to him is fundamental to achieving satisfaction." [4]

Hospital customers are unwilling and sometimes unhappy clients. Healthcare personnel must realize that client services start from the time any client arrives at the hospital entrance and continue until they leave *via* the exit gate. Each personnel can, therefore, enhance or cancel the positive or negative services provided before clients contact physicians or after consulting the doctors. The article "Providing customer support at a critical time: Hospital customer service" rightly captures under "A different approach" the import of customer services in a hospital setting when it states, "Hospital staff are not typically thought of as customer service providers. But in reality, there are many similarities between them and other, more traditional customer service agents. People visiting hospitals require fair treatment, effective communication, and quick responses, just like in other customer service situations. The difference is that people who require hospital customer service are often in the midst of a health crisis, either personally or on behalf of a loved one, and are dealing with intense, emotional scenarios. That is why it is so important to provide customer service that is both efficient and empathetic." [5]

Real patients are not criminals and, when at the gate, security personnel should not treat them as such; they are not dust or dirt that the cleaner sweeps or mops; they are not blood or urine samples that the laboratory scientist works on; they are not drugs that the pharmacist dispenses; they are not the management meetings that managers and heads of department hold; and certainly not the diagnoses that doctors make. We must all realize or remember that we are rendering humanitarian services – no matter how hefty the bill of a private hospital may be or how "affordable" the bill of a government-backed and subsidized service may be. It is when relations like spouses, children, parents, or even colleagues of hospital employees become patients that you see a typical hospital worker switch into the expected normal mode for relating with and attending to a patient. This selectively good (ideally, normal) attitude towards service provision is what should characterize our services to all clients. There is undoubtedly burnout among many healthcare service professionals in developing countries; this, however, should not make us snap at our patients and their relations and treat them as objects as though they are our problems. Clients in the hospital setting can broadly fall under those who receive services from hospitals and those who provide services to hospitals. Those who receive services are the ones just described, while those who provide services include, but are not limited to, contractors who build and maintain structures and equipment and suppliers who deliver equipment and consumables regularly or on a needs basis.

Healthcare personnel* – *Public perception – In developing countries everyone has a perception of healthcare personnel, whether core professionals or support staff. The perception may be right, wrong, or warped. Whatever the perception is, it is important to know that something generated it. Some people hold a perception about a hospital or about its personnel generally or particular personnel even before setting foot on the grounds of the hospital or meeting the workers. This shows how sensitive the work of a medical facility and its personnel is. Of particular note is the not-so-correct impression that people who are outside the healthcare delivery system have about doctors and other hospital workers; many people hold the opinion that hospital workers are rich people but do not realize the amount of effort and sacrifices that hospital workers make. Hospital workers themselves may find that they are stuck in their profession and cannot convince anyone else that they are not who/what the outsider passionately believes that they are. Unfortunately, the hospital worker sometimes shoots themself in the foot by attempting to run the rat race with external professionals. Hospital personnel should resist the temptation of making additional money out of "vulnerable persons" while their perceived "competitors" are making money legitimately out of "goods." The difference is always clear. If such a thing is practiced or encouraged, it breeds animosity towards hospital personnel. From a correct or biased public perception, it is sometimes difficult for the public to agree with and support doctors and other healthcare personnel when they "cry" over one challenge or another.

Organizations and institutions associated with hospitals – There are government organizations or professional bodies that have the responsibility of seeing to it that hospitals in Nigeria work efficiently. Some of these organizations of government include the Ministry of Health at the national and state levels. Hospitals owned by the government, like University Teaching Hospitals, Specialist Hospitals, and Medical Centers report to the Ministry of Health at national levels and hospitals owned by the various state governments report to the various State Ministries of Health. Many sub-national governments also have boards and institutions that go by various names; these manage hospitals under the Ministries of Health. Other institutions have been set up by national governments and they bear various names; in Nigeria, examples are the Medical and Dental Council of Nigeria, various Councils and Boards of specialties like Pharmacy, Nursing, Laboratory science, and Radiography. These apex bodies regulate the practice of medicine, dentistry, and other specialties that are found in the hospital setting.

The Federal Ministry of Health and Social Welfare lists regulatory bodies in the healthcare sector in Nigeria as follows:

- Medical and Dental Council of Nigeria (MDCN)
- Nursing and Midwifery Council of Nigeria (NMCN)
- Medical Rehabilitation Therapist Board (MRTB)
- Radiographers Registration Board of Nigeria (RRBN)
- Optometry and Dispensing Opticians Registration Board of Nigeria (ODORBN)
- Dental Therapists Registration Board of Nigeria (DTRBN)
- Institute of Public Analyst of Nigeria (IPAN)
- Community Health Practitioners Registration Board of Nigeria (CHPRBN)
- Pharmacists Council of Nigeria (PCN)
- Institute of Chartered Chemist of Nigeria (ICCON)
- National Institute of Pharmaceutical Research and Development (NIPRD)
- National Primary Health Care Development Agency (NPHCDA) [6]

Professional bodies are myriad and include the Nigerian Medical Association, Medical and Dental Consultants Association of Nigeria, National Association of Resident Doctors, Association of Nigerian Private Medical Practitioners, National Association of Nursing and Midwifery, Pharmaceutical Society of Nigeria, and unions like Joint Health Sector Union.

The idea behind all these organizations and institutions is to establish and run hospitals, regulate the practice of the various specialties in the healthcare sector, and allow the various practitioners to have special bodies they belong to. The entire thing is to ensure control, discipline, and good practice within acceptable national and international standards. It is, therefore, expected of the various state Ministries of Health to inspect and license all non-government-owned hospitals in their areas of authority and the national Ministry of Health to establish, equip, run and maintain the national government-owned hospitals and receive reports from the managers of those institutions on behalf of the national governments. The regulatory bodies are to ensure that individuals in each of the specialties are properly licensed to practice, keep a record of their professionals, ensure continuing professional development, as well as establish and implement disciplinary measures against professionals who are found wanting. The professional groups seek the welfare of their members and act as pressure groups to get whatever they consider equitable treatment. Unfortunately, there is almost no designated group that represents the clients of medical facilities. Patients should come under national or state Health Insurance Schemes, but there are many that do not come under such schemes due to low coverage in their countries; they come as individuals and pay for services out-of-pocket. Until both patients (clients) and medical institutions (service providers) are adequately represented and protected in the various health insurance schemes in Nigeria and similar developing countries, it will remain difficult to make things work.

When the chips are down, everyone benefits from hospitals in Nigeria working efficiently; conversely, if we do nothing (or not enough) and allow a slide in funding, structure, equipment, function, attitudes, and service provision in hospitals in Nigeria, making hospitals functional and working efficiently will remain a mirage.

CONCLUSION

It is essential that governments, businesses, schools, religious organizations, communities at all levels, and individuals recognize and treat hospitals as integral parts of society. Until that happens, the chances of Nigeria or any other developing country moving forward to the point of actualizing their potential shall remain slim. This is because while Nigeria and these other countries are in the race for development and prosperity, the poor health of their people shall certainly stifle their efforts. Everybody should invest in health, for continuing to do otherwise is nothing less than putting the cart before the horse.

REFERENCES

[1] WHO. Hospitals 2024. Available from: https://www.who.int/health-topics/hospitals#tab=tab_1

[2] CDC. National center for health statistics. Health, United States Hospital 2024. Available from: https://www.cdc.gov/nchs/hus/sources-definitions/hospital.htm

[3] WHO. Healthcare Delivery 2024. Available from: https://eurohealthobservatory.who.int/themes/health-system-functions/health-care-delivery

[4] Hospital Customer Service: A patient-centered care. In: Hospitals: Arab Hospital Magazine Available from: https://hospitalsmagazine.com/hospital-customer-service/

[5] Zendesk. Providing customer support at a critical time: Hospital customer service 2024. Available from: https://www.zendesk.com/service/ticketing-system/hospital-customer-service/

[6] Health regulatory bodies in Nigeria In: federal ministry of health and social welfare. Federal Republic of Nigeria Hospital Services 2024. Available from: https://www.health.gov.ng/Source/27/Hospital-Services

List of Contributors

Emmanuel Kunle Abudu	Department of Pathology, University of Uyo, Uyo, Nigeria
Inyang Ukot	RST Clinics Ltd., Federal Housing Estate, Uyo, Akwa Ibom State, Nigeria
Osahon Enabulele	Department of Family Medicine, University of Benin Teaching Hospital, Benin City, Edo State, Nigeria
OmoOlorun G. Olupona	Bowen University Teaching Hospital, Ogbomos, Oyo, Nigeria
Raphael Sunday Olarewaju	Mother and Child Hospital, Lagos, Nigeria

CHAPTER 1

Functionality and Efficient Services Delivery in Nigerian Hospitals– An Overview

Osahon Enabulele[1,*]

[1] *Department of Family Medicine, University of Benin Teaching Hospital, Benin City, Edo State, Nigeria*

Abstract: It was with great pleasure that this author accepted the book author's request to pen a general view on the title of this important book, **Functionality and Efficient Services Delivery in Nigerian Hospitals**. This title is appropriate and reflects a conscious effort by the author to galvanize efforts towards strengthening much of Africa's health system using the Nigerian health system and its hospitals as a template.

A cursory look at the title of this book may suggest that our hospitals (Nigerian hospitals, in this instance) are not working to deliver the expected efficient and quality healthcare services to their clients and patients. This deduction is similar to what seems like a general public perception that hospitals in Nigeria are not working.[1] Indeed, the poor state of hospitals is said to be one of the factors promoting outward medical tourism, characterized by frequent foreign medical trips by Nigerians, including top political and public office holders.

The above deductions and impressions notwithstanding, it is important to state at the outset that the situation may not be that gloomy, particularly as there are some hospitals in the public and private health sectors of Nigeria, nay Africa, that are still holding their own despite the perennial challenges besetting them. Some watchers may even argue that in the face of the general decay in Nigeria's public institutions, her public health institutions, including her public hospitals, seem to have fared better than some other institutions in the sustenance of their critical responsibility and mandate for healthcare service delivery.

In developing this chapter, the author leveraged their practice experience as a medical doctor and Consultant Family Physician, experiences as a Health and Civil rights activist, involvement in the processes that led to the enactment of Nigeria's National Health Act (NHA), and the practical leadership experiences within health systems at local, state, national, continental, and international levels. This is particularly true, having served as President of the Nigerian Medical Association (2012–2014), President of the Common Wealth Medical Association (2019–2022), and President of the World Medical Association (2022–2023).

[*] **Corresponding author Osahon Enabulele:** Department of Family Medicine, University of Benin Teaching Hospital, Benin City, Edo State, Nigeria; E-mail: osahoncmavp@gmail.com

[#] *Impact Clinics Ltd. has since replaced the former company name RST Clinics Ltd.*

Inyang Ukot (Ed.)

Keywords: Chief medical directors, Federal ministry of health, National health act, NHA-2014, Nigerian medical association, Policymakers, Strikes.

INTRODUCTION

Functionality and efficient service delivery in Nigerian hospitals depend on an understanding of and paying close attention to virtually every word in the title of this book. This chapter commences by describing the word "Hospital." An extrapolation of the definition shows that it is not just a place but what happens in that place, who occupies that space, and for what purpose. For a hospital to exist it means that somebody, a set of people, an organization, or a government must conceive it. This chapter discusses these "conceivers." Since an existing thing or entity does not need creating, it means that the conceiver must be thinking forward. It is this thinking forward that is a problem when it comes to a hospital, groups of hospitals, or a layer of hospitals. When something is right with the "thinking forward," the results will show, and when something is wrong with the "thinking forward," the results will also show. This is where functionality comes in. Functionality must be incorporated into the planning process. Otherwise, it becomes cumbersome or impossible to make practical modifications to achieve functionality if it is not considered, forgotten, or kept in the background. Efficient service delivery dwells mainly onthe human beings in a hospital. Briefly and put simplistically, human beings are the patients and healthcare providers. The fact that a hospital is in existence and is equipped does not translate into efficient service delivery. There will surely be service delivery, but will it be poor, suboptimal, or efficient? The bulk of the responsibility depends on the healthcare providers and much less on the healthcare services beneficiaries (patients). The healthcare providers should be seen as the "powers behind" the existence of the hospitals or hospital system (proprietors, government, investors, *etc.*) and the "direct and indirect operators" who are the healthcare providers who consist of the core healthcare professionals and support personnel, respectively. Patients are very important, though their responsibility is less; they are important because if they do not play their role well, they may either contribute to inefficiency in the delivery of services or complicate it. In Nigerian hospitals, many patients—whether rightly or wrongly—bypass primary healthcare facilities and go directly to teaching hospitals, overwhelming their capacity and negatively affecting the quality of services provided.

Functionality and efficient service delivery in Nigerian hospitals also depend on variables outside the confines of the hospitals and the healthcare delivery system. These are all described not only in this chapter but also in the rest of this instructive book.

Definition of Terms

Before proceeding further, a concise definition of some operative terms is imperative.

Our: The Cambridge English Dictionary defines "Our" as:

(1) Of or belonging to us; (2) Belonging to or connected with us [2].

With the foregoing definition, the focus of this overview is on hospitals located in Nigeria, where I practice as a Consultant Family Physician and served as President of the Nigerian Medical Association (2012–2014).

Hospital: The same Cambridge English Dictionary defines a hospital as a place where people who are ill or injured are treated and taken care of by doctors and nurses [3].

The World Health Organization (WHO) defines a hospital as an establishment that provides short- and long-term medical care consisting of observational, diagnostic, therapeutic, and rehabilitative services for people suffering or suspected to be suffering from a disease or injury and for parturient women. It may or may not also provide services for ambulatory patients on an outpatient basis [4].

The WHO further states that hospitals are reservoirs of critical resources and knowledge that complement and amplify the effectiveness of many other parts of the health system, providing continuous availability of services for acute and complex conditions [5].

It is also important to note that aside from medical service delivery, a hospital may also provide education and training for its staff, health professionals, and students. It may also be involved in the conduct of biomedical research.

Brief Historical Excursion

Global Experience

It is trite knowledge that before the emergence of hospitals, healthcare had always been extended to those in need (especially the sick and injured) in one form or another. Scriptural and historical accounts indicate that early physicians engaged in solo practices and visited the homes of sick ones, where they offered them treatment. In other instances, the sick were treated in the homes of early physicians, in some temples, or make-shift shelters, sometimes located in the fringes/outskirts [6]. Even Hippocrates (the father of modern medicine) and his

Hippocratic doctors were reported to have visited and treated patients in their homes and occasionally performed surgical procedures [6].

Historical records suggest that the earliest hospitals may have existed in ancient Mesopotamia where, towards the end of the 2nd Millennium BC, royal physicians at Assyrian and Babylonian courts cared for ill court singers in elementary hospitals or nursing homes [6].

Precursors of modern-day hospitals were said to have been successively developed through the ages, from the earliest times through the Greco-Roman era, the Christian era, the medieval times, and the Islamic era (particularly during the Golden Age of Islam, which ended in the 13th Century) [6].

The Nigerian Historical Experience

The Nigerian experience, with regard to the evolution of the hospital system and the healthcare system, is not substantially different from the global experience.

Nigerians had always accessed healthcare services in one form or the other before the emergence of modern healthcare services offered by the first group of foreign doctors who accompanied the Portuguese traders that settled in the district of Benin in the second half of the 15th century, precisely in 1472 [7]. Though this modern form of healthcare services and hospital care was initially not extended to the local populations, it was the evangelizing missions of various religious missions that helped to extend modern forms of healthcare to Nigerians through the hospitals they established. It was only in the latter part of the 20th century that the colonial administrators committed to the extension of medical services to Nigeria's local populations through some colonial developmental plans that included the plan for the establishment of hospitals. They were only initially concerned about rendering healthcare services through established military hospitals to their colonial soldiers and their civilian counterparts. This was particularly after World War II [8].

Following the various pre-colonial, colonial, and post-colonial developmental plans, the number and quality of hospitals and other accouterments of Nigeria's health system have been improved upon [9].

Classification of Hospitals

Whereas there are several ways in which hospitals are classified globally, hospitals are generally classified in Nigeria according to their objectives, nature of administration, and the level of care.

According to Objectives

Teaching hospitals, General hospitals, and Specialist hospitals fall under this category.

According to the Nature of Administration

In this class are Public/Government hospitals, Private/Non-governmental hospitals, Faith-based/Mission hospitals, and hospitals owned by voluntary agencies.

According to the level of care

In this class are Primary care hospitals, Secondary care hospitals, and Tertiary care hospitals.

Functions of Hospitals

Though there are various factors that influence the kind of functions carried out by hospitals, they are generally expected to discharge some basic functions such as acute (critical/emergency) and chronic care services as well as out-patient and in-patient care services. These include preventive, diagnostic, curative, and rehabilitative care services.

Some hospitals also offer teaching and educational opportunities to staff, undergraduate, and post-graduate students, as well as research opportunities.

Challenges that Nigerian Hospitals Face

There have been significant developments in some hospitals in Nigeria, even in recent times. These developments notwithstanding, the stark reality is that when placed on a balance, the current story of Nigeria's hospitals is pre-eminently an unpleasant one laced with unattractive performance indicators that fly in the face of local, national, and global expectations.

It is the great worry over the generally doleful state of hospitals in Nigeria, particularly public hospitals, that may have informed the choice of the title of this book, **Functionality and Efficient Services Delivery in Nigerian Hospitals.** It is imperative to identify factors and challenges that may have conspired against the expected growth and development of hospitals in Nigeria, with an emphasis on public hospitals. In this regard, the author wishes to unfurl the following challenges that need to be urgently addressed. The challenges advanced here are by no means exhaustive, but they are critical and significant enough to warrant attention and urgent resolution by relevant stakeholders, stewards of these hospitals, relevant health authorities, and public and political officeholders.

Challenges

Poor Political will and Commitment to the Health of Nigerians

Many Nigerian political and public officeholders at various levels of government seem to lack the political will and commitment required to maximally invest in the development of modern, state-of-the art hospitals and health facilities across Nigeria.

Aside from projecting hospitals in Nigeria as mere consulting clinics during political campaigns, not much happens to fix them after politicians are elected into office. Rather than invest in the development of hospitals and other health facilities in Nigeria, they fly abroad for their healthcare needs, a trend that has increasingly worsened in recent times, with an attendant huge capital flight of over $2 billion [10].

Apart from some efforts made during a previous leadership dispensation to bring about some level of simultaneous upgrade of hospitals across Nigeria, not much has been seen since then.

Another evidence of poor political commitment is the paltry budgetary allocations to hospitals and the health system at federal and state levels, despite universally agreed prescriptions of what should constitute the minimum budget for health. For instance, successive governments in Nigeria have consistently observed the breach of the famous 2001 Abuja declaration of African Heads of State, which prescribed a minimum budgetary allocation of 15% to the health sector [11]. Sadly, in the last 10 years, the average budgetary allocation to Nigeria's health sector has been below 5% [12].

Inadequate Funding

This is one of the critical challenges confronting both public and private hospitals in Nigeria. Poor budgetary allocations to public/government hospitals, in addition to inadequate releases, late releases and sometimes no release of allocated funds, have almost become the norm. These result in a significant negative impact on the capacity of public hospitals to deliver efficient and quality healthcare services to their patients and other clients.

With paltry overhead and capital budgets most times, public hospitals generally find it difficult to develop their infrastructure and achieve their organizational mandates, needs, and expectations of their patients and clients. These budgetary releases are sometimes subject to some political considerations, with some Chief Medical Directors/Medical Directors having to visit the nation's capital, Abuja, to lobby for their releases. There have been instances where some hospitals received less than ten percent (10%) of their required vote for overhead.

The case of private hospitals is worse. Aside from the fact that they receive no form of financial support or subventions from the government, they are faced with poor access to credit, loans, and grants. Even when credits are available, the prohibitive interest rate makes it an unprofitable venture. Many private hospitals are therefore, forced to rely solely on their own limited sources of finance to fund the running and development of their facilities.

Governance and Leadership

Those who framed the extant provisions of the University Teaching Hospitals (Reconstitution of Boards, *etc.*) Act, Cap.U15 L.F.N 2004 prescribed some core attributes, values, and requirements guiding governance and leadership determination in public tertiary hospitals. What has become increasingly glaring in recent years is that these prescriptions, particularly the processes for ascension to leadership in most federal tertiary health institutions and hospitals, have been held hostage by inane and primitive considerations, with merit and other objective considerations thrown overboard. In many instances, the leadership ascension processes have been completely hijacked by external political players and forces, with those that eventually emerge as Chief Executives (Chief Medical Directors/Medical Directors) of these hospitals expressing fidelity to these external players and forces rather than to the hospital and its constituents. This has tended to affect the overall direction and performance of these institutions.

Sometimes, those who emerge as Chief Executives from such flawed and skewed processes, lack the vision, leadership frame, and mindset to inspire the constituents towards the attainment of organizational objectives and goals. At times, some of these Chief Executives see their ascension to such leadership positions as an avenue and opportunity to conquer their perceived enemies. Ludicrously, some even become laws unto themselves with the adoption of adversarial approaches in their engagements with staff, unions, and associations. These are negative traits and attributes unexpected of the leaders and managers of such health-sensitive and delicate institutions.

As commonly said, leadership is everything. If the leadership and governance processes are corrupted, what then can be expected from such Chief Executives or hospitals?

In the private sector, the leadership most times is solely driven by the owners of the hospital, except in cases of public limited liability hospitals and hospitals run by religious institutions.

In solely driven hospitals, a major challenge is the absence of strategic leadership and organizational plans, including leadership succession plans. This evident deficit has been the undoing of most private hospitals, as their sustained growth, development, and prospects are invariably affected negatively. This partly explains why hitherto prosperous private hospitals go into extinction when their sole owners pass on.

Another factor is the absence or non-enforcement or poor implementation of policy or legal frameworks and guidelines for health, including the National Health Act enacted in the year 2014. More often than not, most of these frameworks, guidelines, and legal prescriptions are observed in breach, thus affecting the quality of healthcare services and the overall functionality of the health system. A good example is the poor implementation of the National Health Act since it came into existence. Aside from the provisions that emplaced the Basic Healthcare Provision Fund (obtained largely from the 1% of the Consolidated Revenue Fund), most other provisions, including the provisions that seek to set better quality standards expected to be maintained by health facilities and technologies, have been observed in the breach.

High Cost of Services

On account of the downturn in the Nigerian economy with the attendant effect on the cost of consumables, materials/equipment required in hospitals, as well as the high tariff on needed hospital equipment, a lot of the existing hospitals (including federal government-controlled tertiary hospitals) are most times pressured to pass on these costs to their clients and patients by way of the increased cost of services provided by the hospital. This can have negative knock-on effects on service utilization and healthcare delivery, as most patients (on account of the high poverty rate in Nigeria) may not be able to access essential services. This, in the long run, may negatively affect the productivity of such hospitals, particularly the quality of services offered by them, as well as the aggregate health and wellbeing of the population they serve.

Human Resources for Health

One glaring challenge being faced by both public and private hospitals in Nigeria is that of human resources for health. This challenge manifests in several ways, including, but not limited to, inadequate number, skill mix, and competencies, as well as the poor orientation and attitude of available staff. It seems to have worsened in recent times on account of the burgeoning phenomenon of brain drain, which is traceable to the defective human resource for health development strategy and plans; this is particularly reflected in the defective staff recruitment and student admission policies of most hospitals, payment of uncompetitive wages in the face of a recessed economy, insecurity, poor working conditions and conditions of service, festering inter-professional disharmony, inadequate investment in training and retraining, and poor orientation given to staff.

It is now commonplace to see hospitals recruiting less than their declared staff vacancy, resulting in fewer personnel providing services. Consequences are complications such as overcrowding and long patient waiting times, frequent breakdowns and burnout of the few available hospital staff, with an overall negative impact on the quality of service delivery and the level of patient satisfaction.

Inter-professional Disharmony

Perhaps one of the things that has bedeviled Nigeria's public health sector and the hospitals therein for over a decade now is what this author prefers to call inter-professional "beauty contest." This is what some might call inter-professional disharmony or inter-professional rivalry amongst the various health professionals and health professional groups/associations/unions in Nigeria's public health care sector.

This unfortunate debacle, which is virtually non-existent in the private health sector, is traceable to a "beauty contest" for turf, professional power and status, relevance, economic rewards, authority, and leadership.

This intriguing phenomenon which has adversely affected the quality of healthcare delivery in Nigeria's public hospitals, could have been easily nipped in the bud through the implementation of basic de-politicized administrative mechanisms, but was unfortunately allowed to fester until the then President of Nigeria, Dr. Goodluck Ebele Jonathan, GCFR, declared it as an emergency, followed by the setting up of the Alhaji Yayale-Ahmed Committee of Experts on Inter-professional harmony in the public health sector.

Unfortunately, the disharmony still lingers despite efforts by some groups and associations, particularly the Nigerian Medical Association, to resolve the matter.

As President of the Nigerian Medical Association (NMA), the author initiated several efforts in this direction, including paying visits to other health professional associations and regulatory bodies, and attending annual conferences of other health professional bodies. Our executive of NMA also organized NMA's first-ever National Health Summit in 2013 (Monday, January 20 – Saturday, January 27, 2013) in Asaba, Delta State. There was a dedicated period for a panel session that featured frank discussions by the leaders and representatives of various professional bodies in the health sector, on ways of resolving inter-professional disharmony in Nigeria's public health sector. The gains realized from these efforts are however, yet to yield the desired dividends.

Strike Actions

Another issue that has become a sad commentary in the annals of Nigeria's healthcare sector has to do with the spate of strike actions in the health sector.

While this author urges all stakeholders to join hands to address this phenomenon in our healthcare sector altruistically, it is regrettable to note that it may be difficult to eliminate strike actions that Nigerian workers/employees, including medical doctors/dentists, and other health workers, embark on. This is due to factors which include the low level and low rate of socio-economic development of Nigeria, inadequate provision for the welfare of workers, and poor working conditions. Other considerations are the ever-increasing needs of medical doctors, dentists and other health workers by the State and its agents and the inter-professional "beauty contest" amongst health professionals in the public health sector.

Other triggers of strike actions include insincere, unjust and unfaithful implementation of government directives and circulars by Ministries, Departments, and Agencies (MDAs) of government, as well as the poor management of incipient and emerging workplace conflicts sometimes traceable to indiscriminate creation of new job categories with poor and blurred job descriptions.

From this author's vantage position and experience as a player and leader in the health sector, particularly as one who earnestly tried to address the malaise of industrial actions in the health sector through the organization of the very first NMA National Health Summit, he can unequivocally state that, frequently, it is the insensitive, reactionary, and lack-luster dispositions of Government and its agents in the MDAs, that contribute significantly to the spate of strike actions in the health sector.

The NMA executive council members tried, during this author's tenure as President of NMA, to introduce a new era of constructive engagement between the Government and Nigerian doctors. This was a part of the resolutions of the NMA 1st National Health Summit to project a paradigm shift in the relationship between the Government (and its agents) and Nigerian doctors/NMA. The NMA did not make satisfactory progress; this was because, at every turn, we found the government and its agents unable to brace up to the new paradigm of engagement that they labored hard to project. They preferred to rely on their age-long, outdated approach towards the resolution of conflicts in the health sector.

This unsavory experience explains the author's concern and sadness when some privileged political and public officers at local, state, and federal levels, and other employers of labor, put the blame on Nigerian medical doctors, dentists, and health workers; this is even when it is evident that they deliberately or inadvertently pushed the latter to embark on avoidable industrial actions.

Why, for example, should a Government owe its health professionals/health workers, in some cases, many months' salary, and still expect them to offer satisfactory healthcare services in public hospitals? Why do they throw up the "No Work No Pay" Policy even when they provided the triggers for the strike actions, and ought to observe a "No Pay No Work" Policy?

Insecurity of Staff

Insecurity of hospital workers has become a major challenge with a negative impact on sustained service delivery. This situation, which is connected with the level of insecurity and poverty in Nigeria and dysfunctional health facilities/systems, manifests in various ways, including kidnapping of medical doctors and other hospital workers, robbery activities inside hospitals, damage to health facilities/hospitals by insurgents, and in extreme cases, murder of hospital staff.

Aside from these, the insecurity of staff has also been heightened by the increasing spate of violence against medical doctors and other health workers by patients and their relatives, as well as the perpetuation of oppressive acts against subordinates in the workplace.

The apprehension over the rising spate of insecurity in hospitals and the entire country is one of the major factors propelling the brain drain phenomenon.

Obsolete and Substandard Infrastructure and Equipment

Most of Nigeria's public and private hospitals lack modern, standard, state-of-the-art infrastructure and equipment. This is worsened by the virtual lack of maintenance culture such that even when modern health infrastructure and equipment are provided, they soon deteriorate due to a lack of regular/periodic maintenance of such equipment and facilities.

Recommendations on How to Make Nigerian Hospitals Functional and Efficient

Having identified some of the fundamental challenges, the author hereby proffers the following recommendations and strategic options for repositioning our hospitals:

Improved Political Will and Commitment

One of the major requirements that need to be satisfied in the task of making our hospitals work is the generation and guarantee of improved political will and commitment to the sustained growth and development of Nigeria's hospitals at all levels. Both federal and state governments must commit themselves to greater investment in public hospitals within their jurisdictions. This commitment should not only be exhibited during their electoral campaigns but, more importantly, during their tenures as elected political officeholders. They must see to it that not only is there appropriate budgeting for health with adequate capital and recurrent expenditures, timely releases of these budgetary allocations to hospitals should also be ensured.

Additionally, they should commit themselves to the implementation of Section 46 of the National Health Act which seeks to restrict the use of taxpayers' resources for sponsorship of foreign medical travel by political and public office holders [13].

Political and public office holders should be committed to the utilization of hospitals and health facilities within their jurisdictions in the country whenever they need to access healthcare services, as this will not only inspire confidence in these facilities but also ensure they are regularly maintained and brought up to standard for use by clients and patients.

Comprehensive Audit, Needs Assessment, and Overhaul

The conduct of a comprehensive audit and needs assessment of hospitals in Nigeria is imperative. This is to ensure that private and public hospitals that do not meet acceptable national and global standards are completely overhauled, upgraded, and re-accredited. It is important that the regularity of such a comprehensive audit and needs assessment be well defined and preferably made a policy or legal prescription.

Infrastructural and Equipment Upgrade

To bring most of Nigeria's public and private hospitals to acceptable infrastructural and equipment levels, there is an urgent need for government at all levels, as well as owners of private hospitals, to consciously embark on massive infrastructural and equipment upgrade, with a clearly defined maintenance policy and culture put in place.

Additionally, the federal government should completely eliminate or review the import tariffs on medical/hospital infrastructure, equipment, and technologies downwards.

Funding

To guarantee sustained provision of quality health care services by both public and private hospitals, very innovative and impactful funding models have to be developed.

For government/public hospitals, there has to be substantial improvement in their budgetary allocations, with timely releases guaranteed.

Efforts must be made to close the yawning gap in the recurrent and capital allocations of most hospitals. Additionally, the managers of the various hospitals must look inwards to generate funding/financing initiatives without putting additional costs on the services offered to clients/patients.

As part of efforts to attract more funds, hospitals should be encouraged to go public by registering as public limited liability companies, but with enough safety valves put on the ground.

Establishment of a Health and Hospital Development Intervention Fund (HHDIF)/Health Bank

In recognition of the poor economic state of Nigeria with almost eclipse of the middle class, coupled with the prohibitive bank interest rates and difficulties experienced by medical entrepreneurs in accessing credit facilities, I had in the course of leading a delegation of the Nigerian Medical Association on a visit to the then President of Nigeria, Dr. Goodluck Ebele Jonathan, GCFR, proposed the establishment of a Health and Hospital Development Intervention Fund (HHDIF). This was in response to what I consider an infrastructural and equipment crisis in our hospitals. Consequently, there remains the need to create a pool of intervention funds to assist medical entrepreneurs and managers of public and private hospitals, health facilities, establishments, and technologies with grants. Additionally, banks should provide bearable single-digit interest rate loans on a long-term basis for the sole purpose of upgrading hospital facilities, equipment, and technologies to international standards.

Though President Goodluck Ebele Jonathan had expressed his government's endorsement and approval of the proposal [14] it is unfortunate that the government could not establish the HHDIF before that administration's exit in 2015. This author is hopeful that current efforts to reenergize the proposal legislatively, albeit renamed "Health bank," will come to fruition.

Human Resources for Health

The deficit in human resources for health, which is persistent in both public and private hospitals, can be addressed through the following:

- Regular staffing audits to ascertain the staffing needs of hospitals, particularly in terms of numbers, attitudes, skill content, and competencies.
- Regular and dynamic staff recruitment in response to the outcome of hospital staff audit. The recruitment should be based on merit rather than native or tribal considerations.

The current bureaucratic requirement of involving all forms of MDAs and the Federal Character Commission in the staff recruitment process of public hospitals needs to be reviewed as it seems to have outlived its usefulness. Indeed, the application of the "Nigerian factor" seems to have been worsened by the involvement of these bodies, coupled with the undue delay of the results of staff interviews under the guise of processing the results through the Federal Character Commission, the Federal Civil Service Commission, and the Budget Office.

To drive the point home, there is the case of a particular federal tertiary/teaching hospital in Nigeria where the results of staff recruitment interviews got released over eight months after conducting the interview, but not without the pressure of an industrial action declared to press for the release of the results. This is totally unacceptable.

- Provision of competitive wages, good welfare packages, and other incentives.
- Provision of good working conditions and conditions of service.
- Regular training and retraining of employees in order to put them on the competitive edge.
- Regular staff orientation and re-orientation.

Leadership and Governance

There is an urgent need for the institution of leadership and governance reforms in our public hospitals.

The process for selecting the chief executives of these hospitals should be made transparent, inclusive, and participatory. In the selection and appointment of the

Chief Medical Directors/Medical Directors of these hospitals, merit should be accorded utmost priority and consideration rather than the common resort to political, native, and ethnic considerations/interests. The eventual appointees must have the right leadership attributes and disposition, the right managerial competences and integrity, a clear view and understanding of their mandates, and other job requirements before they are appointed by the government to superintend over these hospitals.

For the federal health institutions, it will be rewarding for the government to review the current practice of two-term tenures for Chief Medical Directors/Medical Directors, with a paradigm shift to a single, 5-year tenure as is currently practiced in Nigerian Universities. This will help to address the bitter and unhealthy political struggles that most times characterize the quest for leadership positions in these institutions, with the attendant untoward effects. This paradigm shift will also create an opportunity for fresh managerial ideas to be brought on board.

Sincere efforts should also be made to fully operationalize all extant health policy and legal frameworks, including the provisions of the National Health Act.

Institution of Effective and Responsive Labor Relations Unit

To better manage all forms of internal and external conflicts, including industrial action by workers, all hospitals should endeavor to put in place a conflict resolution mechanism, through the establishment of a highly equipped, skilled, effective, and responsive labor relations unit. This, in addition to improved responsiveness of hospital management to the welfare and demands of workers, should substantially reduce work stoppages.

Address of Inter-professional Disharmony: The Need for Implementation of the Report of the Alh. Yayale Ahmed Committee of Experts

While it is sad that after spending huge resources to travel around African, European, and American countries in search of solutions to the inter-professional "beauty contest" in Nigeria's public health sector/hospitals, the submitted report of the Alh, Yayale Ahmed-led 11-member Committee of Experts on inter-professional harmony in the public health sector is currently cooling off on the shelves of the Federal Government [15]. This seems to be due to the Federal Government's inertia to implement the committee's recommendations, particularly as they concern job roles and job descriptions.

The author urges the Federal Government of Nigeria to "dust up" (by revisiting) the report of this Committee of Experts. After giving it its due reexamination, implement the sincere and focused recommendations that are aimed at substantially resolving the unfortunate inter-professional rivalry in Nigeria's public health sector.

Other needed interventions include the urgent review of schemes of service to ensure clear definitions of job roles, institutionalization of clinical governance and international best practices, and a renewed commitment by physicians and other health workers to professionalism. There should be a well-defined set of values, behaviors, and relationships that underpin the trust the public has in medical doctors, dentists, and other health professionals.

Public-Private Partnerships (PPPs)

With the long-standing downturn in Nigeria's economy and the chronic underfunding of hospitals in Nigeria, it will be difficult to get hospitals in Nigeria to attain globally acceptable standards, particularly in the areas of infrastructure and equipment, without quality, corruption-free private sector involvement, engagement, and collaboration.

There is, therefore need for increased private sector participation in our public hospitals, preferably through well-thought-out and laid-down public-private partnership agreements that do not put the hospital or its clients/patients at the losing end.

There is also a need to develop mechanisms to guarantee the attainment of the laid down objectives of the PPP arrangements. One such is the establishment of an independent PPP committee to regularly review, monitor, and evaluate these PPPs and other private sector-driven initiatives and collaborations to prevent corruption, conflicts of interest, and overbearing cost of services.

The foregoing notwithstanding, wholesale privatization of Nigeria's public hospitals should be discouraged as it may substantially increase the cost of service provision and deny a vast majority of patients the required access to healthcare services.

Group Private Practice

With specific reference to private hospitals in Nigeria, there is a need for concerted efforts to encourage the establishment of group private practices, whose advantages far outweigh those of the solo practices and sole hospital ownership structures currently prevalent in Nigeria.

The establishment of group private practices will substantially guarantee the survival and sustained performance of private hospitals, as well-defined leadership and ownership succession plans are more likely to be in place than in the case of sole medical directorship.

Clinical Governance

Our hospitals are in dire need of clinical governance to guarantee sustained quality healthcare delivery. The author had, during his tenure as President of the Nigerian Medical Association (2012–2014), established a Clinical Governance Committee (for the very first time in the history of NMA). This was to develop clinical governance frameworks and standard operating protocols. Following this development, the NMA executive members approached the Federal Ministry of Health to advocate the need for hospitals in Nigeria to establish clinical governance units for implementation of the developed clinical governance frameworks.

The author is aware that the Federal Ministry of Health made some efforts in this direction but, like many things in Nigeria, this initiative does not seem to have been sustained, for only a few hospitals are currently practicing clinical governance.

There is a great need for hospitals in Nigeria to be clinically governed with the establishment of clinical governance units where none currently exist and the strengthening of existing units.

Information and Communication Technology (ICT) and Digital Health

Despite the availability of various forms of ICT and digital technologies, uptake by most public and private hospitals in Nigeria is still less than satisfactory.

There is clear evidence that the utilization of digital technologies in the operations of hospitals helps in the effective management of patients' appointment schedules and patients' waiting time, accountability and reduction of corruptive tendencies, health information and data management, research, and other institutional challenges.

It is this author's opinion that hospitals operating in Nigeria in the 21st century must endeavor to consciously seek effective ways of optimizing the inherent benefits and advantages of current and emerging ICT and digital health technologies, including the use of electronic health records (EHR) systems.

Enforcement of Quality Standards, Laws, and Ethical Frameworks

One factor promoting outward medical tourism and poor utilization of services offered by public and private hospitals in Nigeria is the public perception of poor quality and standard of healthcare services offered in hospitals. This is worsened by the burgeoning phenomenon of charlatanism in Nigeria's healthcare sector.

The foregoing was one of the reasons that informed the need for Sections 12 and 13 of the National Health Act, with respect to the need for prescription of quality standards, re-categorization and recertification of hospitals, health establishments and technologies, and which are now required by law to obtain a certificate of standards before they can legally undertake provision of healthcare services. Unfortunately, several years after the enactment of the National Health Act, not much has been done by the relevant health authority to give expression to this fundamental provision of the Act [16].

For clients, patients, and the general public to have renewed confidence in private and public hospitals in Nigeria, improved and sustained efforts must be made to ensure strict adherence by hospitals to prescribed quality standards, laws, regulatory frameworks, and ethical codes. In this regard, the various health authorities at federal, state, and local government levels, health professional regulatory bodies, and professional associations in the health sector have significant roles to play.

The relevant provisions of the National Health Act that concern the prescription and enforcement of quality standards, particularly sections 12, 13, and 14 of the Act, should be made operational as required by law [16].

With improved security and quality standards, as well as national and international accreditation of our hospitals, public confidence in them will be renewed and boosted, with great potential to reverse outward medical tourism.

Reform of Advertisement Laws and Ethical Codes

One of the factors fueling outward medical tourism with its negative impact on utilization and quality service delivery by private and public hospitals in Nigeria is the lack of quality information on the healthcare services and interventions offered by hospitals. This may not be unconnected with the restrictive nature of the extant codes on the advertisement of healthcare services in Nigeria.

There is a need to undertake a holistic reappraisal and reform of the extant advertisement codes and legal frameworks in order to make them more accommodating to the current healthcare market dynamics, particularly with regard to the increasing demands by clients and patients for healthcare information.

Hospitals can also optimize their use of available ICT and digital technologies to expand public access to information on healthcare services that they offer.

CONCLUSION

Functionality and efficient service delivery in Nigerian hospitals is a reality that must be attained. For existing hospitals where specific challenges have been identified, those challenges must be closed without further delay. For hospitals that are in the planning stage, "Functionality and efficient service delivery" must be incorporated *ab initio*. Lingering variables that are outside hospitals and the healthcare delivery system in Nigeria (*e.g.*, power, water, roads, communications, insecurity, *etc.*) should be treated as priorities by the appropriate arms of government.

There may have been some past and present efforts to improve the standards of public and private hospitals in Nigeria; it remains indubitable that most health institutions, health facilities, and hospitals in Nigeria at local, state, and federal levels need rejuvenation, rehabilitation, and upgrade.

To get all our hospitals to modern standards, there is an urgent need to address the several challenges conspiring against their progress. In this regard, a sincere, transparent, and effective implementation of the proposed recommendations is imperative.

REFERENCES

[1] Newspaper P. Inside some of Nigeria's appalling public health centers. 2018. Available from: https://punchng.com/inside-some-nigerias-appalling-public-health-centres/

[2] Dictionary CE. Cambridge english dictionary. Meaning of Our in English. Available from: https://www.google.com/amp/s/dictionary.cambridge.org/amp/english/our

[3] Cambridge english dictionary. Hospital. Available from: https://www.google.com/amp/s/dictionary.cambridge.org/amp/english/hospital

[4] Park JE. Concepts of health and diseases. In: Bhanot B, Ed. Preventive and Social medicine. 22nd ed. Jabalpur 2002; pp. 11-44.

[5] Hospitals. World Health Organization. Available from: https://www.who.int/hospitals/en/

[6] Francois PR, Louise C. The evolution of hospitals from antiquity to the renaissance. Acta Theologica 2010; 26.

[7] Enabulele O. The nigerian health sector: Burning issues and the way forward. A keynote address and special theme lecture delivered at the opening ceremony of the 2015 annual general meeting and scientific conference of edo state branch of nigerian medical association. Irrua, Nigeria. 21st August 2015. Personal Communication 2015.

[8] Enabulele O. Challenges in Nigeria's healthcare delivery system and solutions. A keynote address delivered at the opening ceremony of the Annual week and Symposium of the Health Writers Association of Nigeria (HEWAN). Lagos, Nigeria Personal Communication 2018.

[9] FMoH. Federal Ministry of Health in Nigeria at 50: Championing half a century of sustainable health

development. Abuja: Federal Ministry of Health 2010.

[10] Enabulele O. 'Medical tourism: The implication for an unhealthy economy.' A keynote address delivered at the opening ceremony of the 2017 annual general meeting (AGM) of delta state branch of nigerian medical association (NMA). abraka, nigeria. Personal communication 2017.

[11] World Health Organization. Health systems. The Abuja Declaration: Ten Years on. Available from: https://www.who.int/healthsystems/publications/abuja_declaration/en/

[12] Enabulele O. Universal Health Coverage (UHC): Leaving no one behind. A keynote address delivered at the opening ceremony of the 2018 Physicians' Week of Abia State branch of Nigerian Medical Association (NMA), Umuahia, Nigeria. Personal communication 2018.

[13] National Health Act. Federal Republic of Nigeria Official Gazette 2014. Available from: https://nigeriahealthwatch.com/wp-content/uploads/bsk-pdf-manager/2018/07/01_-Official-Gazette-of-the-National-Health-Act-FGN.pdf

[14] Newspaper V. Jonathan promises special intervention fund to establish more hospitals 2013. Available from: https://www.vanguardngr.com/2013/10/jonathan-promises-special-intervention-fund-establish-hospitals/

[15] Information Nigeria. Jonathan receives Yayale Ahmed Committee Report, Promises to end 'Unhealthy Rivalry' in health sector 2019. Available from: https://www.informationng.com/2014/12/jonathan-receives-yayale-ahmed-cttee-report-promises-to-end-unhealthy-rival-in-health-sector.html

[16] Enabulele O. "Making the National Health Act operational.'' A keynote address delivered at the opening ceremony of the National Executive Council (NEC) meeting of the Nigerian Medical Association. Enugu, Nigeria. Personal Communication 2016.

CHAPTER 2

The Place of Small Hospitals in the Healthcare System

Inyang Ukot[1,*]

[1] *RST Clinics Ltd., Federal Housing Estate, Uyo, Akwa Ibom State, Nigeria*

Abstract: In Nigeria, there are all types of hospitals. The earlier and latter chapters in this book describe hospitals that may be described as small, medium-sized, or large – this attribution is a rough description and uses physical size as the only determinant. The type and level of services that a hospital provides, its location, and the size of its clientele are immaterial as far as the contents of this chapter are concerned. A primary care hospital may occupy large grounds, while some tertiary health care facilities are small in size.

Keywords: Challenges, Client services, Cost of care for patients, Distribution, Encouragement, Financial assistance, Government influence, Investment in hospitals, Leadership, Location, Nigeria, Ownership, Patronage, Payment for services, Physical access, Poor referral network, Power supply, Services, Small hospitals, Sustaining policies, Water supply.

INTRODUCTION

This book chapter, **The Place of Small Hospitals in the Healthcare System,** is not only about one type of hospital but also indirectly a description of the healthcare system in any developing country, using Nigeria as a veritable example. The type, number, ownership, personnel, level of care, and distribution reflect the importance of health and the impact of wealth on the state or nation [1, 2].

In this chapter, the word "Hospital" encompasses basic, small facilities like health posts, maternity homes, health centers, comprehensive health centers, and small hospitals (usually called clinics) that are high-profile, upscale medical facilities. While some of these are strewn across Nigeria, others are typically located in specific parts of the country. It is difficult to write about all types of small

* **Corresponding author Inyang Ukot:** RST Clinics Ltd., Federal Housing Estate, Uyo, Akwa Ibom State, Nigeria; E-mail: inyang.ukot@yahoo.com

Impact Clinics Ltd. has since replaced the former company name RST Clinics Ltd.

hospitals in Nigeria unless an entire book of a reasonable size is devoted to that purpose.

The state of a nation's public healthcare system has a correlation with the wealth of that country and the level of development enjoyed by its citizens and residents [3].

According to the US News and World Report, Canada is the country with the most well-developed public healthcare system, followed by Denmark and Sweden; the UK is sixth and Switzerland tenth. GDP per capita is GDP divided by midyear population. The GDP of Nigeria per capita in 2014 ($3,201) was much better than the figure for 2017 ($1,941.9), which represented a precipitous fall. Nigeria's GDP per capita in 2019 was 2,230 USD; for Canada, for the same year, it was 45,445.610 USD. The nation's GDP per capita has suffered an even worse fate after 2017 for it became $1,621.1 in 2023. The poor performance of this otherwise great country (going by this economic index) is that Nigeria fared worse in 2023 compared with 1981 when its GDP per capita was $2,187.9 [4].

The context in which "Small hospitals" is used in this book is any hospital that is physically smaller than a general hospital and also usually has a personnel strength of not more than fifty; the number of patients that such small hospitals attend is immaterial. They go by various names like clinic, comprehensive health center, health center, health clinic, health post, and maternity home.

These hospitals are, therefore, expected to fit into the healthcare delivery system of any developing country, including Nigeria. What role do they play in the healthcare delivery system in Nigeria? What impact do they make? Is the impact positive or negative [5]?

On the surface, they are the majority of medical facilities in a country like Nigeria, but where are they? Who operates them? Who patronizes them? What services do they render? What challenges do they encounter? What value do they add to peoples' lives and the economy?

Ownership

Statutorily, in Nigeria, public secondary care hospitals belong to State governments and public tertiary hospitals belong to the Federal government. Secondary care medical facilities are general hospitals and their equivalent. Tertiary hospitals are usually university teaching hospitals, but specialist hospitals belong to this group also.

With respect to hospitals discussed in this work, the ownership resides in private persons, groups of persons, communities, and Local governments. Other owners include Christian missions, *e.g.*, NKST church that operates mainly in north-central Nigeria, and government parastatals that render services to their employees, *e.g.*, Central Bank of Nigeria, and manufacturing companies that run industrial clinics on-site.

Nigerian National Petroleum Corporation Ltd. is exceptional in the sense that it does not just own a chain of big hospitals but they are well distributed in the country. In 2020, the Nigerian National Petroleum Corporation (NNPC) indicated its plan to build hospitals in 12 of the 36 States in Nigeria to the tune of N21 billion. These hospitals were to be sited in the six geopolitical zones of the country [6]. In 2022, it was in the news that this national oil corporation was interested in intravenous plant concession. ICRC is the Infrastructure Concession Regulatory Commission. To show the importance of health, the corporation's Medical Services Ltd. Plans to build five specialist hospitals and one intravenous fluid plant – these are to be sited in the six geopolitical zones of Nigeria [7]. So, in Nigeria, ownership of hospitals comes under a wide umbrella. The examples provided in this paragraph show that any individual, group, or organization that is interested in contributing to the healthcare sector in Nigeria would be licensed to do so if they meet the requirements of the licensing body of government and stick to the category of medical facilities they are accredited to operate.

Distribution

The Federal Ministry of Health and Social Welfare in Nigeria lists twenty hospitals as teaching hospitals in Nigeria [8].

However, in 2007, the Federal government tertiary hospitals, which include university teaching hospitals and specialist hospitals, were 151. They represented 0.88% of the hospitals in Nigeria. The State governments owned secondary care hospitals which were 8.11% of the hospitals in the country. Religious organizations owned secondary healthcare facilities, and theirs constituted 1.93% of the hospitals. A couple of Christian missions also own and operate university teaching hospitals. Private hospitals made up 43.20% of the 17,038 hospitals in the country in 2007, closely following the 7,580 hospitals owned by Local governments, which represented 44.41% of hospitals in Nigeria. As of 2024, the Federal Ministry of Health's Health Facility Registry (HFR) indicates that there are 38,813 operational hospitals and clinics in Nigeria [9]. More recent data shows that in Nigeria, the government owns and operates more health facilities (public) than the hospitals owned and operated by the private sector; this is especially true in the northern part of the country. Overall, the ratio is 2:1 (67% against 33%) [10].

In Nigeria, 88% of hospitals are primary health facilities; secondary health facilities account for about 12%; tertiary medical facilities make up just 0.25% [11]. With an overwhelmingly large percentage of medical facilities being primary health facilities, one would expect a lot of emphasis to be placed on them. This expectation would be justified by the fact that this level of medical facility would be accessible and affordable to every Nigerian or everybody who is resident in Nigeria but the practicality is that it is not always so. These challenges are discussed in this chapter, although not exhaustively. The primary health facilities are operated mainly by the level of local governments in Nigeria, but as of the time of writing this chapter, the local government remains the weakest of the three levels of government in Nigeria [12 - 14].

Most small hospitals are primary care facilities, though a number of them render secondary and tertiary health care services. The level and variety of services they offer depend on their location, available equipment, clientele, level of expertise of in-house and external medical personnel, and other professional personnel.

Location

Small hospitals are sited in every local government area (LGA) of Nigeria. Small hospitals in the form of primary health care centers are available in all local government areas, and some of them have at least one in the local government headquarters, while others have additional centers in other villages or clans in the same LGA.

Briefly, the fourth Schedule of the 1999 Constitution of the Federal Republic of Nigeria empowers Local Government Councils (774 of them in the 36 States and the Federal Capital Territory) to carry out functions to ensure efficient primary health care services delivery. The duties include provision and maintenance of health services and environmental sanitation – these are to ensure that they meet the health needs of residents in their communities.

In Lagos State (one of the most populous States in Nigeria), there is a Health Facilities Monitoring and Accreditation Agency (HEFAMAA). It came into existence in March 2006 and has the mandate to monitor both public health facilities and private health facilities. The objective is for all health facilities in Lagos State to be registered and accredited to ensure that they perform their duties to residents of Lagos State efficiently and safely [15].

The Leadership newspaper in 2023 reported that only 25% of the 34,076 Primary Healthcare Centers strewn across the 774 local government areas (LGAs) in Nigeria are functioning. This is despite the Federal Government headed by then President Muhammadu Buhari using the Basic Health Care Provision Fund (BHCPF) to inject 101 billion Naira into 7,600 primary health care (PHC) facilities nationwide in November 2022 [16]. The exchange rate in mid-November 2022 was 441.19 Naira to 1 USD.

As indicated in another chapter in this book, the distribution of these (and other hospital types) may be inequitable. When some of these small hospitals are in a community, that community may not be attractive to healthcare personnel, or the government at the local level may not provide, maintain, or replenish simple tools like stethoscopes and sphygmomanometers for use by healthcare personnel. Sometimes it is the challenge of the unavailability of simple drugs [17, 18].

This is especially true in riverine areas and other communities in remote parts of this large country with a variety of topography. State capitals are usually one of the Local government areas and these have not only small hospitals but also higher levels of hospitals. Many local government areas have one secondary care hospital and small hospitals. Sadly, there are some communities in Nigeria that do not have access to a primary health center; such communities must find some other sources of care when they have health challenges.

Leadership

Well-organized small hospitals are run by doctors, but frequently, they do not have personnel who are doctors at the head; rather, the heads are nursing personnel or community health officers. Of the doctors that head small hospitals, they have a wide range of experience, levels, and areas of specialization. Many doctors have just their first degrees and are general practitioners; they are in the employ of Local governments or State governments. Specialists work in private hospitals as proprietors, medical directors, external consultants, or employees.

Services

Services that small hospitals render are very wide and range from primary through secondary to tertiary health care services. Primary care services are the majority of care that small hospitals offer; this is especially true of public medical facilities. Mission hospitals offer the same services in their outpost health facilities. Private clinics in some villages or small towns in local government areas frequently render primary health care services. Even in major cities, privately-run medical facilities provide primary healthcare services, especially if they are located on the outskirts of such cities. These hospitals at the fringes of populous towns and cities attend to a mixed group of low-income and middle-income earners and their family members [15, 17]. In the upscale parts of State capitals and the Federal capital, private hospitals provide high-profile medical services, with some limiting their services to specific specialties like general surgery, obstetrics and gynecology, pediatrics, dermatology, and cardiology [13]. Other private hospitals provide a mix of primary, secondary, and tertiary health services depending on the need – these hospitals are equipped to render services that they can call in external consultants to provide. Places in Nigeria that have a relatively high density of health clinics of high quality attract other clinics that are of high quality and render qualitative medical services.

Patronage

Small hospitals enjoy patronage based on their location, staffing level, area of specialization, working hours, quality of service delivery, cost of service, reputation, and external looks. Patronage may, therefore, be by clients of all age groups, children alone, pregnant women alone, or according to pathology. As earlier mentioned, the number of patients that a small hospital attends to is immaterial as it does not define the hospital.

Challenges

The challenges are discussed hereunder as: Common challenges, Challenges of private hospitals, Challenges of mission hospitals, and Challenges of government hospitals.

General Challenges

Only two relevant general challenges are addressed here *viz.*: Access and Power supply.

Physical Access

Access (or otherwise) to medical facilities is a challenge to the utilization of the available, though constrained, hospitals in sub-Saharan Africa, including Nigeria. Barriers to obstetric care include lack of ready means of transportation, physical distance between the homes of patients and medical facilities, the excessive amounts of time that patients spend waiting to receive services in many instances, as well as a poor referral system [14].

A further challenge that geographic access poses to patients' utilization of health facilities is the time it takes to reach such hospitals. In Nigeria, especially in rural communities, it is common for distances that should be traversed in 30 minutes to be covered in 3–4 hours; this is usually the case during the rainy season when bad roads become worse. Such roads are full of pot-holes and large irregularly-shaped depressions; they are frequently flooded and many vehicles (both cars and 18-wheelers) break down and block the naturally narrow roads. Some village roads are impassable by cars making motorcycles, tricycles, and bicycles the alternative means for relatively quick, though inconvenient, transportation. Patients who are on such roads may not reach the hospital in time to obtain a good outcome. Matters seem to be worse for residents in riverine areas without small hospitals; to get to the nearest health facility outside their villages or fishing "settlements," they must use manually operated (hand-paddled) wooden boats or speedboats. Such trips could be precarious at night or during bad weather. It, therefore, happens that occasionally the distance may not be significant by road or by water, but travel time may be the challenge. Due to access issues, the small facility does not receive adequate patronage and the patient does not receive the required service.

Power Supply

In Nigeria, all hospitals have the challenge of public power supply in the following areas: timing (erratic), quality (low or fluctuating voltage), or actual black-out. In the latter case, the part of the community where the hospital is located may not have a public power supply for weeks or months due to transformer problems that may be complete breakdown, theft, or vandalism of major parts. It does not matter who owns or operates the health facility – the challenge of providing satisfactory alternative power for an uncertain length of time is a big distraction and an additional high cost. Power-generating plants or smaller units occasionally change from being backup equipment to being the definitive source of power [19, 20].

Any small hospital that determines to offer a reasonably reliable service must have at least two well-maintained power generators of appropriate capacity. Sadly, there are instances that there is fuel shortage on short notice with attendant astronomical increases in the price of petroleum products for reasons that include strain in relations between petroleum workers and government, unpatriotic acts of sabotage of government efforts, or plain desire to maximize profits. Small hospitals hardly have government approval to maintain significant petrol (gasoline) or diesel storage that they could resort to in such times of crises – unfortunately, healthcare facilities do not enjoy any privileges in terms of getting ready access to purchase petroleum products even at additional costs during such crises.

It is of utmost concern that between 2013 [19] and ten years later, 2023 [20] there was no significant improvement in Nigerian health facilities pertaining to public electric power supply. It may also sound disconcerting that the World Health Organization (WHO), in its Fact Sheet of 31 August, 2023 document as a part of its Key Facts on Electricity in health-care facilities that "In low- and lower-middle-income countries of South Asia and sub-Saharan Africa, approximately 12% and 15% of health-care facilities, respectively, have no access to electricity. The energy access challenge is higher for health-care facilities in remote and rural areas." [21]

Challenges of Private Hospitals

Challenges of private hospitals are hereby treated with emphasis placed on hospitals sited in rural and semi-urban areas. The ones that pertain to small private hospitals in large towns, cities, state capitals, and federal capitals are highlighted.

Water Supply

Supply of running water that is potable is a challenge because public water supply is, more often than not, absent. To have this essential ingredient for the provision of optimal medical services consistently, a small private hospital has to sink a borehole and link it to the medical facility. In some parts of Nigeria, this could be a very expensive venture for a small medical facility as accessing the correct aquifer may not be easy – in some parts of the country, a significant distance must be traversed to reach the required depth; in other parts of the same country, the water obtained is contaminated with iron, other elements, or oil. Maintaining a borehole is a problem as technicians may not be available when their attention is needed.

Uroko, as recently as 2017, wrote that "At Zuba Primary Health Centre, in Gwagwalada, Abuja, Nigeria, there is no water supply so staff buy water for hospital use, including washing linen and instruments and flushing toilets. The clinic has been running for roughly 20 years and has 12 staff members who deal with an average of 30 to 40 outpatients each day. It runs antenatal and postnatal clinics, immunisations, laboratory services and services for the prevention of mother-to-child transmission of HIV/AIDS, as well as a delivery unit." [22] It is sad, but of note, that this community is at the fringes of Abuja, the capital of Nigeria and it is just about a one-hour drive to the city center. What, one may ask, happens in villages and remote areas in the far-flung States of Nigeria, especially the relatively poor States in the various geopolitical zones of Nigeria? If government-owned facilities are constrained regarding this basic utility (water), what happens to an individual who desires to (and actually) commits scarce funds to set up a primary health care facility to attend to the poor in such communities, pay taxes to the government, pay all prescribed levies, grapple with a high turnover of employees, and contend with private maintenance technicians who prefer to stay in nearby towns or more distant cities?

In 2021, Abdulmakik O. reported that "Four in five health centres in Nigeria STILL operating without soap or water two years after the global promise." [23]

Pertaining to private medical facilities and their water requirements, Zhema S, Dada AO, in their journal article "The impact and challenges of private health institutions in Wukari Local Government Area from 1972 to 2015," documented that "Lack of power and water supply is a. big issue nationwide and in the study area as well. Sometimes individual *(sic)* take the extra effort of drilling boreholes which eventually runs *(sic)* dry, therefore the hospital management has to buy water from vendors." [24]

Zhema S, Dada AO in their journal article "The impact and challenges of private health institutions in Wukari Local Government Area from 1972 to 2015," indicated that "It is important to emphasize that Wukari have (*sic*) a teeming population with just a single general hospital which is not sufficient for the need of the people, therefore, private hospitals readily filled such lacuna by supplementing the medical needs of the populace (Babarinsa, 2018) [24].

It is of note that Wukari is the headquarters of Wukari Local Government Area in Benue State. Benue State is centrally located in Nigeria and its centrality in terms of geographical location is comparable to Abuja. This means that, like Abuja, Benue State is not north "enough" geographically and it is certainly not south "enough." In Nigeria, the further north you go or the further south you go, there seem to be greater changes in weather, unpredictability of economic challenges, and greater difficulties in meeting water, electricity, transportation, and other amenities that bring comfort to citizens, residents, and visitors. The author chose Wukari as a suitable location to demonstrate averagely the situation regarding private medical facilities and their impact in Nigeria.

Sharing "Turf"

In some communities, a private health facility finds itself having to virtually share turf with long-standing, well-known and accepted non-orthodox health practices and their practitioners. Such new, or relatively new, medical practices have to be not only professionally correct but also correct in managing relationships. Many doctors and entrepreneurs do not feel encouraged to site their hospitals in such places.

Personnel Matters

Recruiting and retaining qualified personnel is a major challenge. In some communities, these personnel may be sparse in numbers or unavailable; some hospitals have had to resort to less-qualified personnel, like making do with "auxiliary nurses" who are barely trained or having to train them to fit the facility's purpose. When qualified personnel are employed, it is easier to get those who are indigenes of, or reside in, the community where the hospital is. Poor commitment and indiscipline could be problems occasionally. Retaining some of such personnel could be another challenge as even when salaries are paid regularly, the young personnel may be interested in returning to school to study and obtain additional qualifications, or they may be interested in other engagements like petty trading and farming alongside their work in the small hospital. Others may have family issues like getting married and receiving calls to attend to spouses or children outside their practice locations.

These personnel are sometimes essential to the success of the hospital and they know it. It is when the doctor in charge of the hospital, other doctors and nurses, and senior non-medical personnel do not understand or speak the local dialect that they really need the local hands; during the consultation, they may be needed to double as interpreters for the doctor, to ensure good communication with patients who may not speak English. In some instances, it becomes difficult to ensure and maintain confidentiality of medical information as some personnel may not abide by the training they received during the orientation period. If this happens, it could bring a negative reputation for the young or even established practice as it may lose patronage.

Equipment and Consumables

Private hospitals usually ensure that they have equipment that is commensurate with the kind of service they render. Consumables are also usually in stock, as they do not want to lose their clients. They may not always have control over the supply of consumables on time, nor do they keep in-house technicians to attend to the maintenance of equipment.

Range of Cases

Being frontline medical practices, these private outfits may not be prepared for the kind of emergency cases that their patients present with, especially at odd hours. Depending on the location, the personnel who are to attend to such cases may not be present, be incomplete, or not be on the facility's personnel list. The facility may not even be equipped to handle such cases and may barely be able to resuscitate patients and refer them safely and promptly. When patients come with "cold" cases, this is not a big challenge as life is not at stake.

Poor Referral Network

Generally, the referral network is poor as it depends on whatever these hospitals create and establish for themselves individually. The doctor in a rural or semi-urban private medical facility must know doctors in the nearest referral center and make calls and write referral letters to be sure that the patient is attended to by the doctors in the unit-on-call for the particular day in the referral hospital. There are instances that on arrival in a referral center, the patient and relations find, to their chagrin, that the same power challenge in the small private hospital is what applies to the general hospital or university teaching hospital at the time. Mobile telephone and Internet services are frequently unreliable in rural areas and semi-urban areas – and the same occasionally applies in state capitals and the federal capital.

Payment for Services

Private hospitals are frequently accused of putting financial considerations at the fore. This happens because of a lack of understanding of how private practice works in Nigeria and similar developing countries. It is difficult to make a patient and relations understand this when it pertains to three areas: Emergency cases with or without surgeries like road traffic accidents and operative delivery for a patient in labor; major surgeries that are not emergency; and crisis periods, *e.g.*, the COVID-19 pandemic lockdown, fuel crisis, communal clashes. Many clients want services to be rendered and payment made later – usually in installments. This out-of-pocket payment for medical services rendered in private hospitals is a big challenge, especially as virtually every private hospital has had cases of delayed payment, incomplete payment, non-payment, and bad debts relating to bills for medical services rendered; it is worse when the patient dies. Until efficient universal health coverage is achieved by the National Health Insurance Scheme, which should be cascaded to the state, regional, and local government levels, both the small private hospitals and their patients will continue to suffer from this shortcoming of uncertainty in payment for services rendered.

Government Influence

Two areas of interest for discussion regarding government influence in private medical practice are regulation of private medical practice and taxes/levies.

Regulation of private medical practice by government does not appear to be adequate in rural areas and semi-urban areas. This is because there are still pockets of practices that appear genuine but are actually not—such as quack practices that remain undetected and undeterred. The fact that their charges are low makes it difficult for genuine and standard practices to be set up in such communities. For the really rural communities, these quack clinics are "better than nothing." People's lives are occasionally put at risk. This author advocates better regulation, accreditation, and monitoring of private practice, especially in rural areas and remotely located communities.

Taxes and levies are a problem for many private practices. The government should know that many private clinics hardly make the kind of profit their officials imagine that they make. Even hospitals that are run by the government can hardly boast of being able to survive for five years without receiving subventions from federal, state, or local governments – yet pay their employees regularly, purchase drugs and equipment, provide water and electricity for themselves, and maintain the facilities, while concomitantly paying heavily to ensure the security of patients, employees, their cars, and the facility and everything in it.

This author believes and recommends that the various layers of government should encourage private hospitals to stay in business and run good services – and there is nothing wrong with the encouragement being in the form of financial assistance from the government to enable hospitals to be established and stay in rural and semi-urban communities. Recognizing the multiple challenges they encounter in doing business, it is difficult to understand why the government would not take private medical practitioners and their practices as partners with the government to achieve the lofty goals of the government to maintain good health for its citizens.

Challenges of Mission (Faith Based) Hospitals

Mission hospitals generally have the mission of rendering high-quality healthcare services to all patients irrespective of age, sex, and religious bent at an affordable cost. They do not have profit as the main driving force, but they do not set up the practices to run at a loss or eventually shut down. That is why most mission hospitals have survived even where some private hospitals have not. This mission is a double-edged sword as what some patients do not expect from private hospitals or government hospitals, they sometimes expect from mission hospitals. This is responsible for some of the challenges that mission hospitals face.

Sustaining Policies

Two policies that appear to be challenges to small hospitals run by mission hospitals are: attendance to all patients and Rendering qualitative services.

How do they maintain the policy of attending to all patients any time they arrive at these medical facilities? For their secondary (and occasionally tertiary) care hospitals, it is not a challenge as these bigger facilities usually have essential/senior personnel living in the hospital compound. Unfortunately, some patients who are familiar with the workings of the bigger mission hospitals expect the same thing in these small hospitals. In the small facilities, patients must stick to the times that the facilities are scheduled to open to clients.

How do they continue rendering qualitative services to their patients? Assistance from individuals and various groups and efficient management of funds coupled with adequate maintenance of equipment see them through this challenge. Such assistance may not be regular; moreover, the resources and assistance go to the headquarters or the regional coordinating offices and that may cause difficulty in satisfactorily distributing it to the network of these small hospitals.

Cost of Care for Patients

Mission hospitals, like every healthcare provider in developing countries, find that an increasing cost of care for patients is a challenge. For many mission hospitals, the fact that they are not putting up new facilities and are maintaining the ones that were well-built has helped them weather this storm. For a long time, they have been used for high-quality, reliable, generic drugs. This allows mission hospitals to make relatively marginal increases in the bills that their patients pay for services rendered in these peripheral hospitals.

Staffing Matters

Mission hospitals have the challenge of paying their staff competitive salaries and other emoluments. This challenge arises mainly from the fact that they do not receive the subventions provided to government hospitals, nor do they charge as much as private hospitals—yet they operate in the same professional and economic environment as both.

Referral of Patients

The challenge they have in referring patients to a secondary or tertiary care hospital is the same as for private hospitals. The advantage that mission hospitals have is that the peripherally located small hospital is not far, time- and distance-wise, from their main hospital; in such cases, the challenge of referral of patients is more easily overcome, all other factors being favorable.

Payment for Services

Despite all efforts to render good medical services at an affordable cost, some patients are obviously indigent; for such patients, a mission hospital's peripheral outlet may be the only hope. This challenge presents itself from time to time.

Challenges of Government Hospitals

As mentioned earlier, even government hospitals suffer from general challenges. The following are the ones that are occasionally found in government hospitals:

Funding

Government hospitals are the only hospitals that can boast of support in terms of funding while at the same time generating revenue internally. Despite this beneficial peculiarity, the funding may be erratic in the sense that the timing of receiving the funds is not always predictable and the purpose for funds received may not be in the hands of the leadership of the small hospitals. These government hospitals of the Federal government, like comprehensive health centers, similar state government-owned hospitals, and the ones owned by local governments, including health centers, *etc.*, may not be the ones to receive priority attention in the disbursement of funds.

Hospital Facilities

In Nigeria, public facilities tend to be large and have initial excellent looks but do not enjoy the desired high level and frequency of maintenance. For this reason, even these small hospitals tend to be large in physical size and occupy relatively large grounds; neither the physical buildings nor the surrounding grounds receive adequate attention consistently. The ones in rural areas suffer more than the ones in state capitals and local government headquarters, as the latter seem to be more visible to the relevant government authorities. Poor maintenance of facilities leads to dilapidation.

Hospital Equipment

The fact that governments' small hospitals are available does not translate to the availability of equipment and medical consumables. When equipment is available, they are not always in a functional state and maintaining, repairing, or replacing them could be problematic. A study showed that though latex examination gloves were available in 77.18% of healthcare facilities, only 68.10% had sphygmomanometers. With respect to drugs, apart from paracetamol and folic acid being available in 74.31%, selected antibiotics, steroids, and antihypertensives did not attain 30% availability [17, 25].

Personnel Matters

It is perhaps because government employees are assured of their employment status that some of them in the peripheral hospitals tend not to take their work as seriously as expected. Some of them engage in poor attendance at work. This manifests as: staying away from work at will, going to work on the days they choose to do so, and late arrival on the days they go to work, as well as early departure despite late arrival. What is described, unfortunately, applies to the heads of some of these small hospitals just as it does to their subordinates. The remoteness of the locations of some of these peripheral small hospitals tends to make some employees desire to get postings in the form of transfers to more attractive locations. Even when these hospitals are near their places of origin, they still want to move further away because of financial pressures from relatives in the village.

Client Services

Client services suffer in many government hospitals, including the small ones. Despite the good intentions of the government in providing healthcare using the vehicle of small hospitals, it is essential for its employees to treat their clients well; doing so would give the latter the confidence to use the facilities repeatedly and recommend them to other prospective patients.

For government hospitals, the facilities and personnel are there, the population is there, but the neglected state of facilities, paucity of equipment and consumables, and poor attitude of the appropriately-qualified staff conspire to work against the intention of government; the result is that patronage is not commensurate with the investment – but the personnel characteristically maintain their employment.

Investment in Hospitals in Nigeria

Foreign investors seem to be interested in big and medium-size hospitals. This author, however, believes that paying additional attention to small hospitals would be an excellent investment, especially if these (and Nigerian) investors chose to have chains of these categories of medical facilities. They would get not only the patient numbers (which are not lacking in Nigeria) but also a wide catchment considering the expanse of land in Nigeria. In a recent ThisDay Newspaper article titled “A Case for Private Sector Investment in Healthcare in Nigeria” the authors stated “...the Nigerian healthcare industry remains an untapped sector. Investments in the healthcare sector may not initially seem as appealing as those in other sectors, such as oil and gas, agriculture, and telecommunications, but a growing urban middle class, expanding internet access, and a well-established distribution network, indicate a promising future for the medical industry.” [26]

Nigeria has not done well in the area of attracting investment in the healthcare industry when compared with countries outside Africa and even other countries within the continent. In 2023, the Federal Government of Nigeria's budgetary allocation for its people's health was 5.75%. This figure, as low as it is, was the most significant allocation for health in Nigeria's history [26]. Aig- Aig-Imoukhuede *et al* posited that "Nigeria lags behind in its health equity investments compared to other African nations. For example, between 2016 and 2022, Egypt, South Africa, Morocco and Kenya received $1.5 billion, $935 million, $615 million and $379 million worth of investments into their respective healthcare industries, outpacing Nigeria, which received just $351 million over the same period." [26] This aberration could be corrected in a short space of time if the appropriate organs of government at various levels focused on addressing it. Nigeria, with its large population, ought not to be attracting less than 25% of what the less populous South Africa rightly deserves currently.

Nigeria has a huge potential investment in the healthcare market but the current constraints are a veritable deterrent. Nigeria has been having a low health care expenditure that is even lower than the average per capita in Africa; in the average in Africa was $186 in 2019, the World Bank reported a paltry $76 for the same year [26].

Investments in the healthcare sector in Nigeria have become a dire need. It is so urgent that the investments must come from every available legitimate and caring source. Angela Onwuzoo of the Punch Newspaper on 17 December 2023 reported that "While countries like Rwanda and South Africa have met the commitment by allocating at least 15 per cent of their total budgets to health, Nigeria is yet to do so and is still far from meeting the target as the country's health sector challenges keep increasing. A review of the budgetary allocation to the health sector in the last 23 years revealed that Nigeria has never met the 15 per cent target agreed upon in the Abuja Declaration as it is still struggling with less than 10 per cent since the declaration." [27]

The article also stated that "Despite the myriad of problems confronting the health sector, especially the japa syndrome, only about five per cent is allocated to the sector in the 2024 appropriation bill." [27] In Nigeria *"japa"* has widely been accepted to mean "getting out" or "emigration."

CONCLUSION

Small hospitals are in the public sector and private sector. The majority of them belong to the public sector. Services rendered in the public sector do not seem to meet the expectations of the various tiers of government that own and run them. In the private sector, ownership and operation of these hospitals are by a wide group – ranging from individual professionals, individual and group investors, and religious bodies, to companies. The small hospitals in the private sector have multiple challenges which many of them have tackled satisfactorily and made significant strides. Outside rendering standard medical services, profit is the primary aim for individuals and investors in the private sector. Religious organizations do not emphasize profit though they are in the private sector. For companies that run industrial or staff clinics, their goal is not to make a profit but a combination of saving costs, intervening early in and solving employees' health challenges, and maintaining or enhancing productivity.

Though health is wealth, the governments of many developing countries still do not allocate adequate funds to, or spend it on, the health sector; Nigeria, the most populous country in Africa, has, over the years, consistently demonstrated this lack of commitment to improving health and economy as it has been allocating single-digit percentage of its budget to health as shown by the N427.3 billion (<8%) budget for health for 2020; this amount translates to allocating N2,000 to each citizen to attend to their health needs for the entire year; in Nigeria (at the time of writing this book) this amount buys one or two loaves of bread – depending on the quality of the bread [28 - 30]. Unfortunately, the lofty goal of allocating at least 15% of their national annual budgets to which Heads of State of African Union countries committed themselves in April 2001 (over 20 years ago) remains a mirage in Africa's most populous country [31, 32].

Small hospitals have a significant role to play in the health sector of any country. The Federal government, in Nigeria's 2020 budget, initially allocated N44.5 billion (N44,498,247,834) for the Basic Health Care Provision Fund (BHCPF) with the aim of improving Primary Health Care (PHC) in the 774 local government areas in the country. The Federal government cut it by 43% to N25.6 billion ($71 million at the time) or approximately 35.5 cents per person for primary health care for the year [33 - 35].

For the governments of developing countries to make significant progress in the near future, an inter-sectoral approach must be adopted. As mentioned in this portion of this book, poor roads and poor road linkage in Nigeria, poor telecommunication, poor water supply, inadequate, poor quality, and epileptic public electricity supply would continue to counter any move (including an increase in funding) to improve healthcare delivery as long as these stumbling blocks are not tackled practically, passionately, and holistically.

With respect to personnel, doctors will continue to migrate from Nigeria even after being trained in-country up to the consultant level. Improved remuneration and other conditions of service have been advocated for doctors and other healthcare personnel [36].

However, as long as there is the absence of good schools in most local government areas, minimal job opportunities for spouses, security threats that extend to the workplace, and paucity of social amenities, highly qualified healthcare personnel will not be attracted to establish or work in small hospitals in rural and semi-urban parts of the country – and these are where functional and affordable ones are desperately needed. A concentration of relatively good facilities and amenities in cities, state capitals, and the federal capital is what pulls many people to these parts of the country, including healthcare personnel. This leads to a skew in the distribution of these personnel. It is common knowledge that many small hospitals that are manned by doctors do not have them during the weekends. The weekends and public holidays are when many personnel who are not on call travel out to the cities to meet their friends and family members and even go to church, clubs, and attend other social gatherings.

One factor that could dramatically and positively change the contribution of small hospitals, irrespective of their ownership or location, is the establishment of a good local network of small hospitals in every state in Nigeria. A national network that would show the register of contacts of referral centers for certain medical conditions that cannot be handled within particular states would be helpful.

In Nigeria we still do not have a dedicated toll-free emergency telephone number *via* any of the mobile telephone service providers for people to call in cases of medical emergencies. This would be helpful, at least in some cases.

Laws in Nigeria pertaining to healthcare should be modified for the good of the people and medical practice. Of note is the law on advertisement. If people get to know what kind and range of services are available in small hospitals in their local government areas or states, they would know where to go when the health needs arise, rather that wasting precious time moving from one hospital to another.

Since small hospitals in rural areas and semi-urban areas are generally not functioning optimally, many patients bypass them and government-owned secondary care hospitals (general hospitals, cottage hospitals) and go to tertiary hospitals like university teaching hospitals and specialist hospitals. These tertiary hospitals are few (usually only one in one State); they have a discouragingly large turnout of patients with primary and secondary healthcare needs. This means that these referral centers are hardly referral hospitals as patients go straight to them from their homes. Everyone's time is wasted and the patients that these tertiary hospitals were meant to attend frequently spend weeks to be able to consult the specialists and months before they can have surgical intervention for cases that require it. Bed spaces are sometimes clogged with patients whose emergency and other in-patient cases could have been addressed earlier in small hospitals with quicker results.

The place of small hospitals in the healthcare system of developing countries is incontrovertible. Countries in Africa and other parts of the developing world must make maximum use of this great resource to achieve the goal of meeting the healthcare needs of their people.

REFERENCES

[1] Travis P, Bennett S, Haines A, *et al.* Overcoming health-systems constraints to achieve the Millennium Development Goals. Lancet 2004; 364(9437): 900-6. [http://dx.doi.org/10.1016/S0140-6736(04)16987-0] [PMID: 15351199]

[2] Ogunbekun I, Ogunbekun A, Orobaton N. Private healthcare in Nigeria: walking the tightrope. Health Policy Plan. Oxford University Press. 1999; 14: pp. (2)174-81.

[3] Bloom D, David C. The health and wealth of nations. Science. 2000; 287: pp. (1)207-9. [http://dx.doi.org/10.1126/science.287.5456.1207]

[4] World Bank national accounts data, and OCD National Accounts data files. GDP per capita (current US$) –Nigeria Available from: https://data.worldbank.org/indicator/NY.GDP.PCAP.CD?locations=NG

[5] Sato R. The impacts of quantity and quality of health clinics on health behaviors and outcomes in Nigeria: analysis of health clinic census data. BMC Health Serv Res 2019; 19(1): 377. [http://dx.doi.org/10.1186/s12913-019-4141-y] [PMID: 31196212]

[6] Olugbode M. NNPC to build N21bn Hospitals in 12 States Available from: https://www.thisdaylive.com/index.php/2020/06/08/nnpc-to-build-n21bn-hospitals-in-12-states/

[7] Yarling M. ICRC receives NNPC delegation over proposed Specialist Hospitals, intravenous plant concession. Available from: https://www.icrc.gov.ng/icrc-receives-nnpc-delegation-over-pro-osed-specialist-hospitals-intravenous-plant-concession/

[8] Federal ministry of health and social welfare. List of all Teaching Hospitals 2024. Available from: https://health.gov.ng/Source/3/Teaching-Hospital-

[9] The federal ministry of health. Nigeria Health Facility Registry (HFR) 2024. Available from: https://hfr.health.gov.ng/statistics/tables

[10] Makinde OA, Sule A, Ayankogbe O, Boone D. Distribution of health facilities in Nigeria: Implications and options for Universal Health Coverage. Int J Health Plann Manage 2018; 33(4): e1179-92. Available from: https://pubmed.ncbi.nlm.nih.gov [http://dx.doi.org/10.1002/hpm.2603] [PMID: 30091473]

[11] Balogun JA. Types and number of healthcare facilities in Nigeria 2016. Available from: https://www.researchgate.net/figure/Types-and-Number-of-Healthcare-Facilities-in-Nigeria_tbl5_317387397

[12] Nwakeze NM, Kandala NB. The spatial distribution of health establishmentsin Nigeria. Afr Popul Stud 2011; 25(2): 2. [http://dx.doi.org/10.11564/25-2-251]

[13] Kyei-Nimakoh M, Carolan-Olah M, McCann TV. Access barriers to obstetric care at health facilities in sub-Saharan Africa—a systematic review. Syst Rev 2017; 6(1): 110.

[http://dx.doi.org/10.1186/s13643-017-0503-x] [PMID: 28587676]

[14] Wong K, Benova L, Campbell O. A look back on how far to walk: Systematic review and meta-analysis of physical access to skilled care for childbirth in Sub-Saharan Africa. [http://dx.doi.org/10.1371/journal.pone.0184432]

[15] Omoleke II. The primary health care services in Nigeria: Constraints to optimal performance. Niger J Med 2005; 14 Available from: https://hefamaa.lagosstate.gov.ng/registration/public-primary-health-centers/

[16] Ibeh R. Only 25% of Nigeria's Primary Healthcare Centres Functioning – Investigation. Leadership 2023. Available from: https://leadership.ng/only-25-of-nigerias-primary-healthcare-centres-functioning-investigation/

[17] Oyekale AS. Assessment of primary health care facilities' service readiness in Nigeria. BMC Health Serv Res 2017; 17(1): 172. [http://dx.doi.org/10.1186/s12913-017-2112-8] [PMID: 28249578]

[18] Obosi J. Health care crisis in Nigeria. Available from: http://wwwjideobosi.blogspot.com/2007/06/health-care-crisis-in-nigeria-when-did.html

[19] Nwanya C, Ekechukwu V. The energy performance of hospital buildings in Nigeria. Int J Technol 2013; 7(1). [http://dx.doi.org/10.14716/ijtech.v7i1.2094]

[20] Nnodim O. Hospitals grounded, patients suffer as erratic power supply worsens mortality rate. 2023. Available from: https://punchng.com/hospitals-grounded-patients-suffer-as-erratic-power-supply-worsens-mortality-rate/

[21] WHO. Key facts: Electricity in health-care facilities. 2023. Available from: https://www.who.int/news-room/fact-sheets/detail/electricity-in-health-care-facilities

[22] Uroko C. How lack of water undermines healthcare delivery, deepens sanitation challenges. 2017. Available from: https://businessday.ng/health/article/lack-water-undermines-healthcare-delivery-deepens-sanitation-challenges-2/

[23] Abdulmakik O. Four in five health centres in Nigeria STILL operating without soap or water two years after global promise. In: WASH Matters (Policy and Practice). WaterAid Nigeria 2021. Available from: https://www.wateraid.org/ng/media/four-in-five-health-centres-in-nigeria-still-operating-without-soap-or-water

[24] Zhema S, Dada AO. The impact and challenges of private health institutions in Wukari Local Government Area from 1972 to 2015. Available from: https://zjpd.com.ng/index.php/zjpd/article/download/28/30/5

[25] Ephraim-Emmanuel BC, Adigwe A, Oyeghe R, Ogaji DST. Quality of health care in Nigeria: a myth or a reality. Int J Res Med Sci 2018; 6(9): 2875-81. Available from: www.msjonline.org [http://dx.doi.org/10.18203/2320-6012.ijrms20183621]

[26] Aig-Imoukhuede E, Ngwoke O. A case for private sector investment in healthcare in Nigeria. Available from: https://www.thisdaylive.com/index.php/2024/08/30/a-case-for-private-se-tor-investment-in- healthcare-in-nigeria/#google_vignette

[27] Onwuzoo A. 23 years after, Nigeria yet to meet 15% health budget. 2023. Available from: https://punchng.com/23-years-after-nigeria-yet-to-meet-15-health-budget/

[28] Olufemi J. Nigeria budgets N2,000 for the Healthcare of each citizen in. 2020. Available from: www.premiumtimesng.com

[29] 2020 Health Budget – Federal Republic of Nigeria. 2020. Available from: https://budgetoffice.gov.ng

[30] Adepoju P. A breakdown of Nigeria's 2020 budget for health. 2020. Available from: http://www.healthnews.ng

[31] Abuja Declaration ten years after – World Health Organization. Available from: https://www.who.int

[32] Nigeria Health Watch. 2011. Available from: http://www.nigeriahealthwatch.com

[33] Carsten P, Eboh C. Nigeria proposes steep basic healthcare budget cuts despite coronavirus. Available from: https://www.reuters.com

[34] Egba L. The problem with Nigeria's proposed healthcare budget cuts. Available from: http://www.nairametrics.com

[35] Folorunsho-Francis A. Health workers condemn reduction of 2020 health budget by 50%. 2020. Available from: http://www.healthwise.punchng.co

[36] Vujicic M, Zurn P, Diallo K, Adams O, Dal Poz MR. The role of wages in the migration of health care professionals from developing countries. Hum Resour Health 2004; 2(1): 3. [http://dx.doi.org/10.1186/1478-4491-2-3] [PMID: 15115549]

CHAPTER 3

Efficient Human Resources Management in Hospitals

Inyang Ukot[1,*]

[1] *RST Clinics Ltd., Federal Housing Estate, Uyo, Akwa Ibom State, Nigeria*

Abstract: In a typical hospital, nearly everything of significant interest—both living and non-living—relates to humans. The non-living things include the building (if it is a small hospital) or the buildings (if the medical facility is a large hospital at one site or a chain of hospitals in multiple sites). The other constituents of non-living things are the moveable, and installed and immovable equipment of diverse sizes and numbers. Living things are usually considered plants and animals. Plants could be a problem and could also be of great aesthetic value in the hospital setting, as this book shows in some of its chapters. Human beings come under the animal kingdom classification and are considered to be at the top of the ladder in that kingdom. Non-human animals are part of human existence, but they are not considered in this book as the medicine that applies to animals is veterinary medicine. In a characteristic hospital of any size, the consideration or focus is humankind.

This book is about human beings who are unwell and need to be given attention by other human beings (and gradually assisted by robots) to achieve restoration of health, prevention of disease, or promotion of health. In summary, one set of human beings needs help; another set of human beings provides help.

Keywords: Administration, Human resource management, Staffing, Workforce diversity.

INTRODUCTION

It is interesting on the one hand and incomprehensible on the other hand that some people who look at a hospital "from the outside" do not realize that hospitals, particularly the large ones, consist of one of the most diverse sets of employees and service providers. Having worked with a multinational-cum-global oil company and one of the largest banks in Nigeria with established presence in various parts of the world, this author is convinced that the diversity that is found among workers in a hospital is something that should be held dearly and positively beneficial for the employers, employees, patients, and in community a hospital is located.

* **Corresponding author Inyang Ukot:** RST Clinics Ltd., Federal Housing Estate, Uyo, Akwa Ibom State, Nigeria; E-mail: inyang.ukot@yahoo.com

Impact Clinics Ltd. has since replaced the former company name RST Clinics Ltd.

What we find in Nigeria is that even the government at the three established levels fails to make use of the talents and potential of these remarkable people. In the private sector, the same pattern is applicable with significant exceptions in the oil industry.

The diversity and importance of human resources in a hospital can be simplified as follows:

- Direct healthcare professionals – These include, but are not limited to, physicians, pharmacists, nurses, radiographers, laboratory scientists, physiotherapists, occupational therapists, and phlebotomists.
- Indirect but essential support professionals – These are hospital administrators, lawyers, accountants, internal auditors, security experts, *ad infinitum.*
- Broad support personnel – There may be individuals or personnel of third-party contract firms. Personnel in this category are security personnel, and technical personnel like plumbers, electricians, horticulturists, carpenters, roofers, and more.

Understanding this wide range of top, middle-level, and lower-level professionals and personnel is especially important but exceedingly difficult. This is partly attributable to the fact that in many public hospitals, the usual yardstick of importance is what this author would simply call "the paycheck." The value of an employee's paycheck may cause at least two problems: a) It makes an employee feel superior to another employee with less on the paycheck; b) It makes an employer disregard the importance of the low-paid employees. Sometimes, it is not the employer but the employer's representative (or high-level employee like the medical director, group medical director, director of finance, executive director – human resources) who choose to create an unbridgeable gap between the high-ups and "the rest." Where this occurs, managing the human resources of a hospital could be the caterpillar that gradually eats the "leaves" of the hospital, or the pest that attacks the "roots" or "stem" of the hospital. It is by choice that this author is using non-human resources terms in this Introduction so hereby promptly explains leaves, roots, and stem. The "leaves" symbolize any hospital that has grown enough to develop leaves but not enough to produce fruits. The people who matter in handling employee issues may feel that the hospital "business" has flourished because of the satisfactory performance in terms of the financial standing – but they are wrong. The "stem" refers to the visible robustness of the establishment. In Nigeria, this is occasionally a façade and the proprietors of the highly physically visible hospital feel deceived when they send out adverts and are inundated with responses from prospective applicants. In Nigeria, the unemployment rate is remarkably high and continues to rise [1]. According to the Nigeria Economic Summit Group (NESG), globally, Nigeria, with a combined unemployment and inflation rate of 36.9% in the first quarter of 2024, competes very favorably with the worst in terms of misery indices [1]. In Nigeria, less than 10 of the available opportunities are in the formal sector. This means that more than seventy percent of currently employed people hold jobs that are ipso facto vulnerable jobs [1]. How does it feel when today you leave your home for work and in about three months you are jobless, promptly back to the unemployment market? The situation is so bad that when they are paid, they are paid less and the working conditions are inconducive – there are main instances that there are no toilets attached to some workplaces and working hours could be unjustifiably long; these are features of the informal sector. Is it, therefore, surprising that when a job vacancy is posted for ten employees in any place of work that offers some stability in employment status, five hundred or more applicants may apply?

Employees in the informal sector often work without the protection or support of formal structures and benefits, or receive only minimal coverage [2]. The worker finds themselves in a quandary. Do they accept a job that is inherently dangerous, with little or no prospects, very fickle, with many other equally disadvantaged persons seeking similar jobs, or wait and hope to get a job in the formal sector that may equally not assure them of satisfactory or regular remuneration?

The rest of Chapter 3 is devoted to a brief presentation of the following topics; it contains the principles and practices of human resource management applicable in Nigeria currently, with some examples of the situation in the past.

Employment

In Nigeria, it is uncommon for a young university or college graduate to obtain an offer of employment within the first five years after graduation. A generation ago (and slightly earlier), it was possible for a graduate to have an offer of employment in the final year of school. This was so for many doctors and the vacancies were waiting to be filled. Commencing the one year internship (called "housemanship" in Nigeria) was mandatory and some students chose to travel abroad for a holiday before returning to take up the appointment. The process was bereft of any bureaucratic bottlenecks. For other graduates who did not require any internship, life was easier and faster, as they started with the compulsory National Youth Service Corps (NYSC) immediately after graduation. So, for a typical graduate from a tertiary school educational institution, the first employment was assured. Today that is not the case. Some doctors wait to have an opening for months before they can start their pre-registration service that statutorily lasts for one year employment (not from graduation date but from the date that the graduate receives an offer of employment). It, therefore, happens that some privileged or "lucky" doctors finish that first year of employment while some of their classmates are just starting or others are mid-way of the the program. It must be noted that this compulsory year service-cum-practical training occurs only in hospitals that are accredited. Regarding the NYSC program, one could be sure of when the program would start and when it would end; these days, it is when a graduate receives "call up", the person leaves for the orientation program, obtains posting to the place of primary assignment in the State the graduate is posted to and serves out the rest of the "service year." For some graduates, this is not a smooth "first employment" experience for weeks may be spent attempting to "change the posting" to a favorable place of work. The initial "primary place of assignment (PPA)" may be the one to "reject" the "corps member." The system, therefore, ingrains a sense of apathy, unseriousness, lack of respect for time, and other negative tendencies in many young Nigerian graduates. Many graduates testify that the NYSC work experience was the only experience that they had after leaving the "four walls" of a Nigerian university. This is how many Nigerian graduates join other Nigerians who did not have the opportunity to experience tertiary education in Nigeria or outside Nigeria. Going through the Internet for experiences of recent members of NYSC, however, seems to show that the consensus is that it was a positive experience for them. Of the many posts on the Internet regarding the NYSC year, the most recent (dated 2024) ended with this quote: "I believe the NYSC, like many things in life, is what you make of it. It can be a year of growth and adventure, or it can be a year of frustration and stagnation. I also believe the choice should be yours to make." [3] Other reports show that the situation after the NYSC is a concern to many Nigerians. In July 2023, Nigeria's House of Representatives asked relevant ministries in the country to "allow graduates to find employment opportunities." [4] It is doubtful that this request has been followed through, even though it came from this legislative organ of the Federal Government of Nigeria. A young blogger in her post gave useful suggestions to NYSC members on how to position themselves for opportunities to get employment or to create employment for themselves. The suggestions are building soft skills, acquiring additional certifications, and exploring content creation, among others [5]. The purpose of, and approach to, the sub-heading on employment is to show how critical the first couple of years of a young person's life are, as they can shape the future of most Nigerian youths. Many did not think of anything other than obtaining a secure job in the formal sector of the economy, retiring after active service years, and enjoying their retirement years and benefits. Few are cut out for adroitly handling the vagaries of self-employment in Nigeria, where even the so called "secure" jobs have proved unable to live to their name or description.

Leaving the Unemployment Pool; Joining the Workforce

The next step for most young people is to leave the burgeoning unemployment pool and join the workforce. This author breaks down the process into the following:

- Standing out from the crowd – If a pin could identify a good (or the best) in a haystack of job applicants, would it be attracted to you as one (or the only one)?
- Applying for jobs – Not just one effort or to just one potential employer. Filling online forms and providing only the relevant requested information or writing applications professionally.
- Preparing for interviews – Researching the prospective employer.
- The employment interview – Expect some questions; prepare for unexpected questions. Prepare an answer to the question "Do you have any questions for us?"– this question, if asked, is at the end of the interview when the interviewee's confidence would have become boosted or flattened.
- The job offer – Study it; understand the details. Be wary of shallow letters.
- Prerequisite after job offer – You may need to leave your comfort zone. A thorough employer will incorporate free-to-new-employee pre-employment medical examination.
- Assuming duty – First impressions do matter – your time for assumption (first day at work), your dressing, your composure and level of confidence, your interaction with your manager and colleagues, and your short meeting with the CEO if your employment is at a level that requires this personal first meeting.
- Keeping the job – Qualification for the job is different from qualification to keep the job.

Above is an abridgement of the considerations of the prospective employee – and, incidentally, what a potential employer seeks.

The rest of this Chapter briefly addresses some of the core functions of the human resources management (HRM) division, department, or unit. In the hospital setting, it is usually a department or unit. In a large organization, like the major oil companies in Nigeria, they may be called a division of the organization – and HR plays a vital role in the functioning of the entire organization. By whatever name it goes by, HR should tell every employee "Welcome" and "Goodbye" and everything in between. "Goodbye" may be bitter or sweet – the sweet is during the retirement party and the bitter is termination as early as within the probationary period [6]. The HR team is usually headed by a manager, but it could be held by a supervisor, a general manager, or an executive director. This team is so professional that, in this author's opinion, they are the quintessential "politicians" and "ambassadors" of the company. They represent the interests of the company (in this case, the hospital) and represent the interests of the workforce too. They are the best team that understands both the employer and employee. It may be surprising that the HR team does not have to be deeply knowledgeable about the core technical work that goes on in any organization, but they know how to straddle between every employer (and their representatives) and every organization's workforce (and their representatives). How they are able to do this remains an enigma. In 1996 while working as the next to the head of the medical department in one of the largest banks in Nigeria, there was a "misunderstanding" between the staff union and the top management of the bank. One morning I was at work early and my consulting room door was thrown ajar and here walked boldly into the consulting room about five angry bank employees. They angrily asked for my colleague and I, smilingly told them that I had just resumed for the day and we had not met. They disbelieved me. Although they were junior in the system, their lead was very blunt and told me "Doctor, we did not come here to play with you. If you do not tell us where he is, we shall throw you out of this large window!" Indeed, the window was large enough to throw anybody down with ease. Since it was technically the fifth floor, the effect of such a drop can easily be imagined. Yours truly stopped smiling and knew that I was in a predicament. One of them told their leader, "Let us leave him alone; he is not part of this issue." I eventually realized that the union leaders believed that the medical department leadership was not fully in support of them and what they agitated for but believed that we secretly aligned with the decision makers who were really our patients. They did not understand the ethics of medical practice or the boundaries of our work as specified by this major bank. All this took place in the head office on Lagos Island. Who cool-headedly waded into this matter and resolved the "dispute" with top management? The Human Resources department team of the bank! This author has gone through "the archives" of his mind to exemplify the fact that while doctors and the medical department are known to save lives, the HR department saves jobs, lives, families, and businesses!

Recruitment

The HR department is responsible for the recruitment process, which involves at least the following:

- Internal and external advertisement of the job opening(s).
- Screening the applications.
- Creating a shortlist of potential interviewees.
- Invitation to the interview – this may be one day or be well spaced out.
- Selection of the prospective employee.
- Sending out offer letters to the candidates at the top of the list.

- Sending out alternative letters to the next candidate(s) should one or more of the elite candidates decline the offer.
- Liaising with the medicine (and/or occupational health) department to arrange pre-employment medical examinations to assess fitness for employment on health grounds and keeping a baseline record of every new employee's health status.
- Welcoming the new employee(s) – this may be by a circular in the hospital.
- Introducing the new employee(s) to their departmental heads.
- Performing in-processing that allows the new employee to have a record in the organization – in this case, the hospital or hospital group.
- Providing the new employee with a company photo identification (ID) with a unique employee number. This number should not be transferable or re-issuable. This process may be in liaison with the security department.

Orientation

Onboarding an employee incorporates an orientation that is general and may be performed by the HR department designated members of staff only. Another stage of orientation may involve a specific orientation for the new employee to have not only a general feel of the company (hospital) but also get the opportunity to familiarize themselves with the department or unit they are assigned to. A new employee will do well to ask as many questions as possible to get a proper understanding of the working environment job description.

Retention

It is inconceivable that a hospital would go through the abridged processes described so far and not be interested in the retention of the engaged employee. The new employee must not be cocky when they realize that they were "the best from the crowd of applicants." This is because every employee gets watched. There is no need to mention who does the watching as it may be misleading just as it may belie the level of comprehensiveness. What is watched is more precise and includes the employee's suitability, capability, and teamwork skills. Inasmuch as the hospital wants to retain every employee, this is impractical because the feedback that the HR department receives may indicate that an employee should be let go within the probationary period. This is usually ninety days to six months [7]. If it is longer than that, some new employees may feel uncomfortable with the long time it takes to attain full employee status. This is because it is more difficult for a person to "hide" the negatives in 90 days than in 365 days, and as indicated, an employee who is found unsuitable for a position may be let go of the probationary period mentioned in the letter of offer of employment (and the employee would have accepted). The HR department would have documented this acceptance letter before allowing the employee to resume duty. Unsure employees are sometimes terrified by the possibility of losing their jobs with little or no notice [8].

Briefly, other HR functions are applicable to employees who have proved their mettle and stand a chance of keeping their jobs in the hospital. The functions that the HR department anchors or coordinates in liaison with the technical or professional departments and their units are:

- Trainings
- Appraisals
- Promotions
- Transfers
- Disciplinary actions
- Separations (beyond the probationary period)
- Retirements

CONCLUSION

The conclusion of this Chapter comes as two pieces of advice *viz.*:

- If your hospital can afford an HR Department, please do, and if you do, let at least the leadership of this department be well sought out and be on board before you fully commence business. If you do not take this route, you are really "putting the cart before the horse" and you may have cause to go through the discomfort of only partially succeeding in mending the faults that could have been avoided.
- If you can neither afford an HR Department, Unit, nor trained HR personnel, you must have a working knowledge of the principles and practices of the HR function, otherwise, your hospital could be walking through an invisible "forest" that ends at the edge of a cliff. The result is predictably unpleasant.

This author observes that a good Human Resources Management department has a way of selecting and maintaining a team of human management "diplomats." Over the years, it is still baffling to this writer how the team consistently wades through muddy waters and stormy seas and still gets the job done to the general satisfaction of the employees and the employers. They do this best when the proprietors of a hospital give a free hand to function and remember that HR departments are not rubber stamps of the business owners.

REFERENCES

[1] NESG. Nigeria's unemployment rate increased further in 2024Q1. Available from: https://nesgroup.org/blog/Nigeria%E2%80%99s-unemployment-rate-increased-further-in-2024Q1#:~:text=

[2] ILO. Informal economy. Available from: https://www.ilo.org/projects-and-partnerships/projects/partnership-improving-prospects-forcibly-displaced-persons-and-host/themes/informal-economy#:~:text=

[3] The NYSC experience in Nigeria: A year of service and self-discovery. Available from: https://www.splintertalk.io/@vickiee/the-nysc-experience-in-nigeria

[4] Akpan S. Reps ask employers to retain corps members for one year after NYSC. The Nation 2023. Available from: https://www.thecable.ng/reps-asks-employers-to-retain-corps-members-for-one-year-after-nysc/

[5] Orji C. How to Get a Permanent Job after Your NYSC Year. L Geopay 2024.

[6] What is a probationary period and how does it work? In: Oyster 2024. Available from: https://www.oysterhr.com/library/how-long-should-a-probationary-period-be

[7] Darwin Box. Probationary Periods - Meaning & Definition. Available from: https://explore.darwinbox.com/hr-glossary/probationary-period

[8] Craig W. What is a probation period and why are they important? In: Safe HR. Available from: https://www.safe-hr.com/insights/blog/what-is-a-probation-period/

CHAPTER 4

Functional Structures for Efficient Service Delivery: Considerations for the Management of Health Facilities

Inyang Ukot[1,*]

[1] *RST Clinics Ltd., Federal Housing Estate, Uyo, Akwa Ibom State, Nigeria*

Abstract: The development and management of hospital facilities should follow a systematic process, including, at a minimum, conceptualization, planning, design, construction, maintenance, provision for growth, and security considerations. This chapter is designed to cover these aspects. The contents are not exhaustive but are adequate to demonstrate considerations, challenges, and successes in achieving functional and efficient medical facilities management.

Keywords: Design medical infrastructure, Facilities management, Hospital planning.

INTRODUCTION

This chapter explores the challenges and successes in achieving functional and efficient medical facilities in Nigeria. The stories are actual stories of what has happened, used to happen, and is still happening in hospitals in Nigeria. The stories of many hospitals are discussed in this chapter to highlight successes and offer suggestions for enhancing the functionality of the medical facilities. The aim is not to criticize but to acknowledge that, while no facility is designed to fail from the outset, some may encounter flaws either at inception or during their operational lifecycle. Every medical facility in Nigeria is welcome, and more should be built and operated efficiently. The population of Nigeria is projected to continue growing, as it has yet to reach a plateau; this means that there shall be an increase in the pressure that is placed on medical facilities in Nigeria. These hospitals, as described in other chapters of this book, are varied and could be government-owned hospitals, faith-based hospitals, company hospitals, educational institutions, medical facilities, or private hospitals. Whatever the ownership is, a hospital may provide primary, secondary, or tertiary healthcare services (sometimes offering just the first two levels, and at other times, all three).

* **Corresponding author Inyang Ukot:** RST Clinics Ltd., Federal Housing Estate, Uyo, Akwa Ibom State, Nigeria; E-mail: inyang.ukot@yahoo.com

Impact Clinics Ltd. has since replaced the former company name RST Clinics Ltd.

Conceptualization

A physical structure is the product of the mind. The mind may be that of an individual or the mind of a group of people. If more than one person is involved, it may be that they are a couple, a family, friends, business partners, a company, an institution or an organ/arm of government, people of the same religious faith, and others. The more people involved in conceptualization, the more time and input are involved. When it is one person, there is usually a shorter time because numerous meetings that two or more people would necessitate would be obviated. In either case, there are challenges. One of the challenges with many people is the possibility that one or more of them could be dominant "voices" and may not listen to the opinion of even the majority, but one of the advantages is that all aspects of the matter in question are considered and the result stands a good chance of success. With one person, there may be the challenge of "myopia" that makes the individual not see "beyond their nose." This tends to happen when this individual is the embodiment of everything about the concept, especially if the person is the financier in toto.

When it comes to a hospital, it is good for a doctor to be involved but it could be dangerous if that doctor does not listen to anybody but believes that being the professional and having the funds, they need no input from external sources. In this unfortunate situation, the result shows up like a sore thumb in the future, and onlookers and clients would wonder how and why that is the case. The reason is that conceptualization is really the unseen, intangible, and most important foundation of a medical facility and, indeed, any physical structure.

Planning

In this chapter, a simple approach was adopted to planning as outlined in *Business Jargon* [1]. With regard to planning a medical facility, the components of planning extracted from this interesting write-up are goal-oriented and futuristic. These two are considered the sine qua non. There must be a goal. What are you trying to build? Are you building it because you have so much money or because you have funds limitations? Do you have a clear idea of the hospital in your mind, or is the idea foggy or in flux? In terms of goal, do you know where you are going with this hospital? Where are you taking patients, employees, and third parties? Is your planning in consonance with the reality of the goal in your mind, or is the planning tangential to the goal? Regarding futuristic, are you living in "the now" only, or do you think about the future? Which is more important to you, now or the future? Are you sure that your planning for this medical facility is based on you, or is it based on another person or other people? Specifically, are you certain that you are not on a "competition trip" with your medical school classmates or juniors? Is this planning for something that will last or will certainly fade away? Are you aware that many businesses do not survive beyond five years? Is your planning to put you in this class of the majority of businesses or in the elite class of the dogged businesses?

Design

The design of a building starts with having lucidity regarding the purpose of the structure; in this case, a hospital. It must be noted that the term "hospital" can refer to vastly different entities, much like the word "animal" can apply to both an ant and an elephant. So, which one are you asking the architect to design for you (the client)? Do you have any idea of your own that could be incorporated into this design? If you do, do you want to dictate everything regarding the design? Or do you extricate yourself (or yourselves) from the design and simply tell the architect, "Design a ten-bed hospital for me?" or "Design a seventy-five-bed hospital for us?" Which architect have you chosen, or are you considering choosing for this design? What experience does this professional have regarding designing hospitals? Are you engaging them because they are a family member, church member, club member, or some other sentimental reason? Is it because this architect successfully designed an office that caught your attention? Remember, a hospital is not an office, residential building, restaurant, or hotel; it encapsulates all of them.

Briefly stated, your proposed hospital must be designed to attend to the following: entrances, exits, water (and appropriate plumbing), power (and the best and most convenient outlets as sockets and lighting), heating, ventilation, and air conditioning (HVAC) [2]. Other important considerations are ease of movement, like corridors, verandas, ramps, and restrooms, among other features. A hospital is not a place designed for use by healthy people (although the healthy people are engaged as employees and third parties), but principally by the unwell, who must not be exposed to further hazards and inconveniences like uneven floors, multiple steps, absence of elevators/lifts/escalators where they should be incorporated at the design phase. The design of your hospital, therefore, constitutes an approved set of documents that detail the architectural, engineering, and technical characteristics of the building-to-be.

Construction

As briefly stated earlier in this chapter, a hospital, especially a large one, is a peculiar building and should be treated as such ab initio. The construction of a medical facility entails unique challenges. Apart from incorporating safety controls for everybody, particularly patients, the unseen challenge of infection must not be ignored but controlled or reduced significantly. Many hospital equipment, like the ones in the operating rooms, laboratories, and drugs in the pharmacy, should be stored within the temperature ranges specified by their manufacturers [3]. Achieving this goal in hospitals in Nigeria is a herculean task, as 24-hour electricity is the standard. Even hospitals that are located in parts of the country's capital that are served by band A public electricity supply still do not have an uninterrupted power supply, although the unit price for electricity they consume in this band is much higher than the other bands. An additional budget must be included during construction to have a seamless installation of high-profile solar units to make up for the deficit; the alternative of constructing houses to keep heavy-duty electricity power units or plants tends to be cheaper than solar installation in the short run but is uneconomical on the long run. This is discussed in other chapters of this book, but this insertion suffices to indicate that the best time to consider it is during the construction phase of the hospital development.

For infection control, establishing and maintaining negative pressure rooms is important because they "contain harmful particles by making sure that air flows into the room rather than out, using sealed HVAC systems to maintain the correct pressure levels" [3].

Maintenance

The USAID document with the title "Primary Health Care Project" defines maintenance as "A group of sustainable technical and administrative activities, which aim to preserve devices and equipment and restore them to the normal functional condition for them to perform the required tasks properly and reduce cost and time effectively." When applied to the entire medical facility, the definition would conveniently replace "devices and equipment," and the meaning would be more comprehensive and elaborate [4].

In this chapter, maintenance is considered as a whole and specific. The USAID document is used as it provides an abridgement that this chapter requires [4].

The 2013 document pertains to Primary Health Care Clinics in Iraq. It classifies maintenance into planned maintenance and unplanned maintenance. From the very names/adjectives given to these two types of maintenance, the planned one should be the preferred one. Planned maintenance is further described as being either regular maintenance or corrective maintenance. Unplanned maintenance, on the other hand, involves emergency situations or becomes a tool during breakdowns [4]. Another way of classifying or describing maintenance is *inter alia*: reactive maintenance, preventive maintenance, and proactive maintenance. Using just these three, their advisability level is rated progressively higher, starting from reactive maintenance.

Pertaining to Nigeria, the findings of Ebekozien *et al.* reported in their work titled "Maintenance of Public Hospital Buildings in Nigeria: An Assessment of Current Practices and Policy Options" had shortcomings in the areas of budget and funds disbursement, specialized workforce, and a defined program, and schedules of action [5]. The effects include but are not limited to inadequacy in meeting statutory requirements (with no consequences for non-compliance), the avoidable but unfortunate overlooking of incorporating maintenance into the construction phase of the construction, and the owners and top management of public hospitals not appreciating the significance of maintenance as a key factor in sustenance and improvement of their medical facilities [5].

As mentioned previously, maintenance is the crux of a medical facility; this is irrespective of the size, location, or cost of the entire medical facility. The tendency would be that if attention were given to the maintenance of the whole facility, attention to the parts thereof and the equipment, furniture, and furnishing within the "four walls" of every part of the medical facility would get the same benefit. On the other side, a tale of woes is the inevitable experience of consigning maintenance to irrelevance in the scheme of things in any hospital (public or private), and it would be a dangerous slide. Many hospitals in Nigeria have suffered this unfortunate experience and the structure and equipment become liabilities rather than assets. A few hospitals actually become abandoned over the years. In Borno State in the northeast geopolitical zone of Nigeria, two communities (Waddiya and Malamari) have unused healthcare centers, and this situation has pushed the already under-served residents into "deadly health crises" [6].

In a case reminiscent of what is documented above, Governor Sani of Kaduna State (north-central geopolitical zone) of Nigeria acknowledged the abandonment of nearly three dozen general hospitals in this pivotal state. It must be noted that, in the Nigerian healthcare setting, general hospitals lie in between the primary healthcare centers and the teaching hospitals that provide primary healthcare only and tertiary healthcare statutorily, respectively. Most patients should have access to general hospitals, but what are the implications when a significant number of these facilities are abandoned? This abandonment is not just of the physical structures but also the grounds and the contents within the abandoned physical facilities [7].

To explain the pervasiveness of the phenomenon of hospital abandonment, the next example is from the southwest geopolitical zone of Nigeria. In this example from Ogun State, the story is not about an old, dilapidated structure but a construction project abandonment of a humongous "250-bed medical facility built by the immediate past governor of the state, Senator Ibikunle Amosun, in the Oke

Mosan area " [8]. At the time of making the report in Punch News, neither the previous nor the current government had completed the hospital project. The author of that article employed vivid imagery by including the fact that this potentially high-profile, well-intentioned medical facility had become a "hospital where termites and others are the patients" at the time of the report [8]. Herein lies one of the enigmatic experiences in Nigeria – abandoned hospital projects, even at the point of installation of equipment, but usually at various points of construction prior to equipping the facilities.

Provision for Growth

The conclusion from the work of Kapologwe *et al.* on facilities development and upgradation in Tanzania [9] is immensely helpful in summarizing this key area in the functionality of and efficient service delivery in Nigerian medical facilities. It can be concluded that "there has been improvement in the physical status of primary health facilities as a result of constructions, upgrading and equipping the facilities to offer safe surgery and related diagnostic services" [9]. This means that if Nigeria were to follow this pattern judiciously, there would not be the challenge of constructing hospitals in an unplanned and un-strategic fashion, as will be demonstrated in the ten examples in the second part of this chapter. Kapologwe *et al.* further documented that "despite the achievements, there is still a high demand for good physical statuses and functioning of primary health facilities with the capacity to offer essential and safe surgical services in the country, which is also an important strategy towards achieving UHC" [9]. UHC is an acronym for Universal Health Coverage; it is one of the goals for health care delivery in Nigeria. Nigeria has more hospitals and used to have more personnel than Tanzania. It is instructive that although Tanzania has made noteworthy progress in the construction and upgrade of its medical facilities, it deems these successes suboptimal, inclusive of the functionality of its medical facilities, an important aspect that this book addresses regarding hospitals in Nigeria. Even if an upgrade of a medical facility is not in the sphere of physical expansion, it should be in purpose and quality of services rendered. However, functionality and efficient service delivery cannot occur in a vacuum. They must take place in a physical facility where human beings are able to function and where other human beings can receive the services with some modicum of respect and humaneness; the employees, patients, and other people who have to do one thing or the other in a medical facility should be able to do confirm these benefits.

Safety Considerations

The author of this work had a nine-year stint working for ExxonMobil in Nigeria's Niger Delta. In those years, he was exposed to top-notch safety precautions and implementations. This global company recognized, implemented, and embodied the principle of "safety" in its operations. This is one of the unforgettable and irreplaceable benefits that the author, as a senior staff physician, received during that period. It must be stated here that the lessons learned have impacted him in every area of his personal, family, and business life. Considering the aspect of safety considerations in a medical facility, the owners, designers, and operators must know that without safety, their facility and business are at risk. The hospital building, the perimeter fencing, the entrances and exits, the alert system, the plumbing system, the electrical system, and the close-circuit television (CCTV) system must be in place safety-purposed and functional. Even the flooring and housekeeping should be treated as safety hazards as they could pose sources of falls to children and older patients [10]. Fire safety and firefighting capabilities, emergency access of the ambulances, and many more features must be consiered while building a hospital. These features are even more pertinent when the medical facility is planned to be (and eventually becomes) a high-rise building. Safety and satisfactory functionality go hand in hand [11]. Small, medium, and large hospitals must have designated, accessible, and readily identifiable muster points that not only the employees but also all patients, patients' relatives, contractors, and visitors must be made aware of and become familiar with.

Security Considerations

There is a tendency to treat security and safety as synonyms; this is especially so because, in many write-ups, they are placed and addressed side by side. However, this sub-heading separates security from the sub-heading on safety. Security can be easily understood as external threats to your business/workplace, person, family, or property (or further, like your neighborhood, community, state, or country). In this chapter, the security considerations are about the property (physical building and every physical thing within and outside the building but within the perimeter of the total property legally owned by the medical facility).

Among the ten possible and known security threats in a hospital that Accutech Healthcare Security Solutions indicated in a post on their website are personal, hospital property like drugs, patients' private and confidential medical information, drugs, client elopement, theft or kidnap of patients like pediatric patients, and violence in the hospital setting [12]. All these are experiences in hospitals in Nigeria and will be incorporated into the ten examples that are discussed in the first part of the chapter.

Examples of Aspects of Functional and Efficient Facilities Management of Hospitals in Nigeria

These are the stories of specific hospitals where the author of this chapter has worked or has been remarkably familiar. Some will be named, but others will be treated with anonymity. The ones that are mentioned by name are mentioned because the author knows the status of the information as of the time of writing in 2024. The others are not mentioned because there may be significant positive changes, or the balance of change may tilt towards the unsavory side. Since it is good practice to maintain confidentiality, in the latter cases, specificity regarding names and locations shall be excluded from their stories.

St. Luke's Hospital, Anua Offot, Uyo, Akwa Ibom State, Nigeria

This hospital is where the author was born, indicating that the hospital is much older than seventy years old. Some hospitals do not survive beyond ten years, and other forms of businesses fizzle out by five to seven years. This catholic mission hospital has a popularity that extends beyond Akwa Ibom State. It has proved itself beyond any reasonable doubt to be a functional hospital that has rendered efficient services to the populace for decades. This hospital occupies adequate grounds; the grounds are properly asphalted where there are roads, and the spaces beyond the road have beautiful, well-maintained grass, plants with flowers, and trees that provide shade and a sense of seriousness of purpose and originality in planning. The hospital has well-spaced buildings that exhibit age stratification, which is expected of an institution that has maintained the old, developed the new, and continues to construct without any evidence of cramped spaces. The facilities are appropriate for where there are supposed to be bungalows; where the purpose requires multiple floors, they are erected to meet the purpose. One of the most attractive features of this "ancient" yet "modern" secondary healthcare facility is the absence of dilapidation. It is quite common in Nigeria to find hospitals that are less than half the age of St. Luke's Hospital and have dilapidation "written all over them." Credit must be given to the management of this large hospital, the owners of the hospital, the donors (if any), the employees, and the patients. This author includes the patients and their relatives because he is familiar with the fact that some of the poor state of the structures of some hospitals and their utilities and part of the sorry state of the grounds (where grounds still exist) is a contribution by patients and their relatives. They do not seem to respect any rules (written or unwritten) and care only about their welfare. The looks of St. Luke's Hospital may be therapeutic to patients who love nature, beauty, and order.

Figs. (**1** to **14**) present various aspects of this hospital, and the images are as current as late 2024.

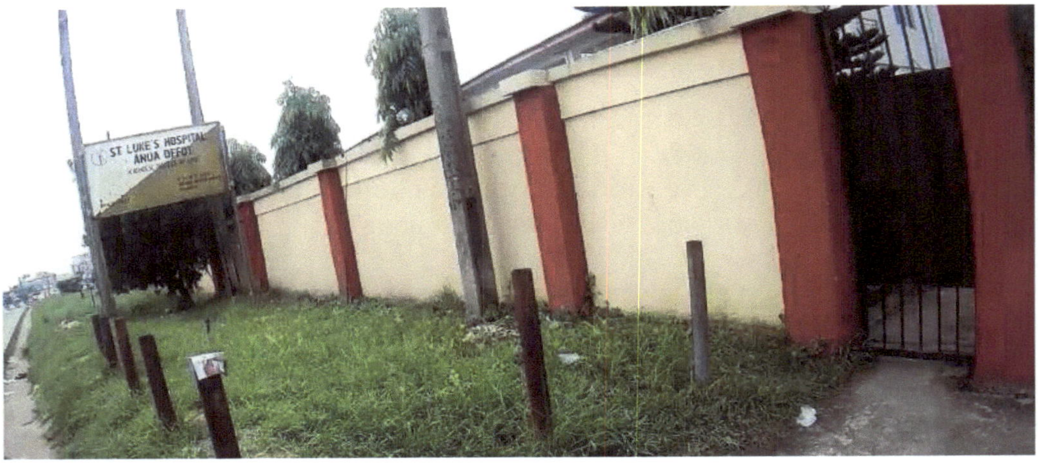

Fig. (1). The signboard of the hospital.

This is the front of the hospital; metal barriers are installed to alert passersby not to walk on and through the well-maintained grass. The hospital is on a major road in Uyo. Uyo is the capital city of Akwa Ibom State.

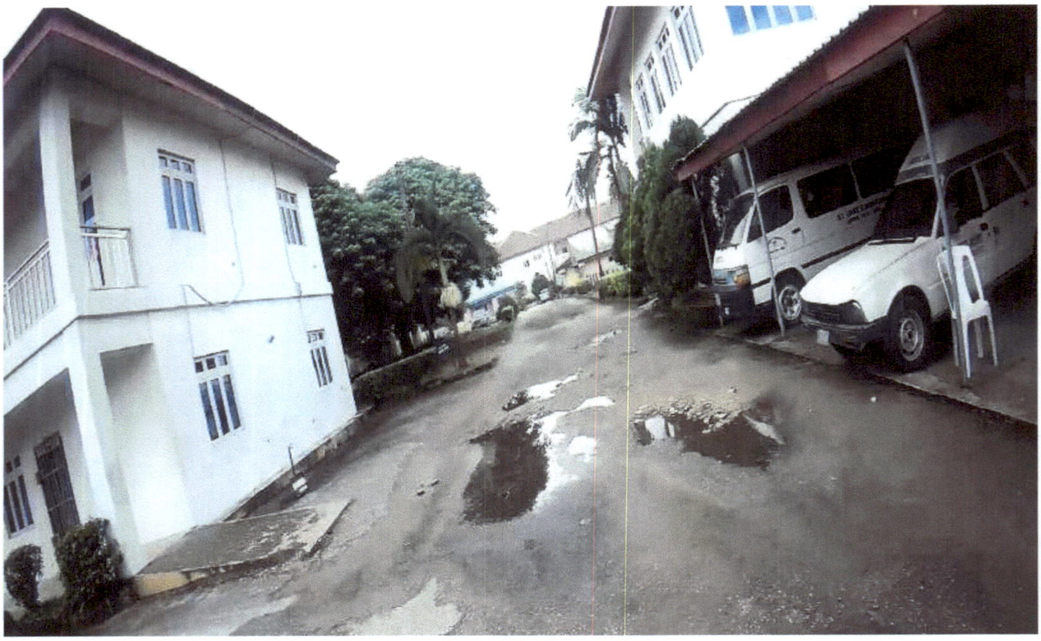

Fig. (2). This photograph shows a road within the hospital.

There is some water after rainfall, as shown, but there are no serious potholes. There are no speed breakers (called and known locally as "bumps") on this road.

The order and orderliness of this hospital are shown by the absence of vehicles parked on both sides of the road within the compound. The two hospital vehicles are in their designated parking spots. The Peugeot 505 is one of the hospital's ambulances. The building on the left has a ramp that allows patients with mobility challenges to be wheeled into that building. This detail, basic as it is, is lacking in some hospitals in Nigeria.

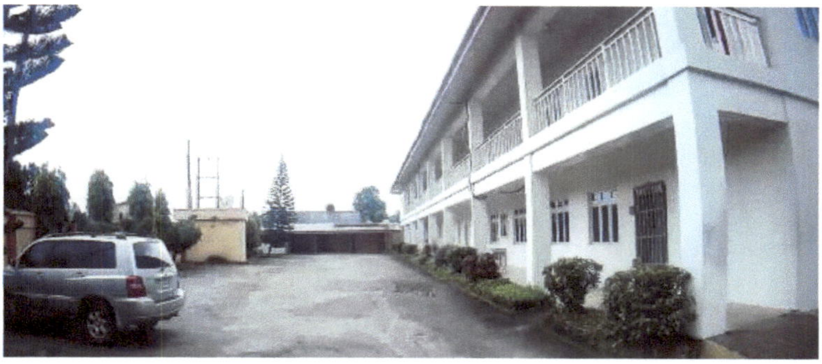

Fig. (3). The state of maintenance of the white building on the right is commendable.

The green area in front of the building is well-kept. There is no piece of paper, an empty can of drink, an empty plastic glass of water, or a discarded sachet of water on this road.

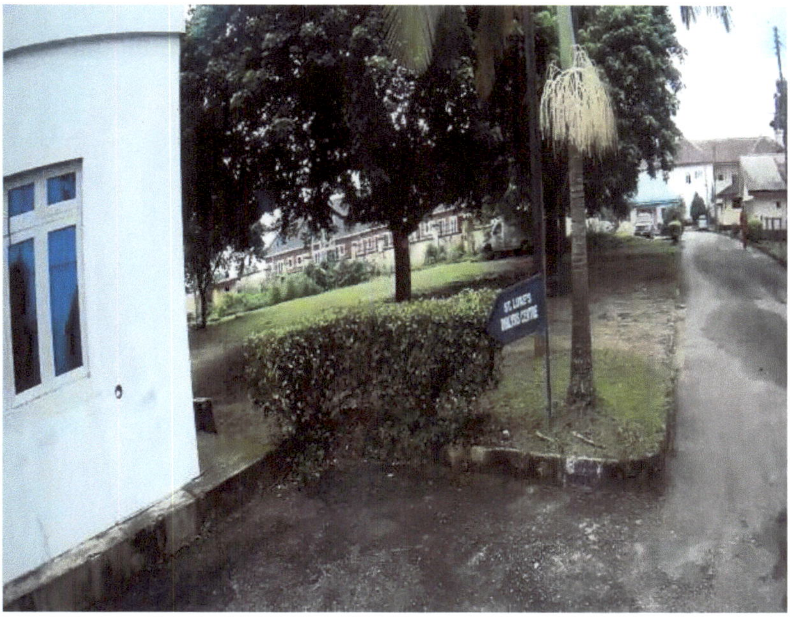

Fig. (4). Signage in St. Luke's Hospital.

Signage is one of the features that are lacking in some hospitals. This hospital pays close attention to that. The inscription on this signage with an arrow design indicates "St. Luke's Dialysis Centre." Every hospital, particularly the busy ones, should copy this good example of providing signage to direct patients and relatives.

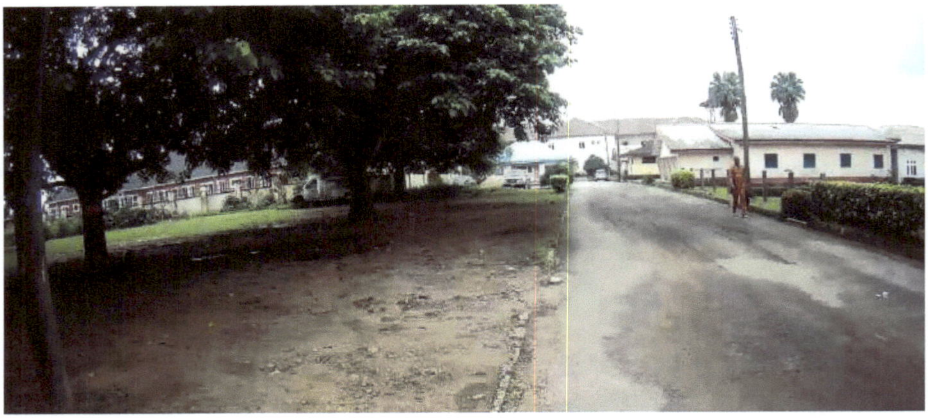

Fig. (5). Purpose-planted trees.

One scarcely finds purpose-planted trees in the compounds of large hospitals in Nigeria. The usual situation is much of the space occupied by buildings with a good percentage of them uncompleted for many years or even abandoned. In St. Luke's Hospital, this view shows well-spaced buildings in addition to areas for trees.

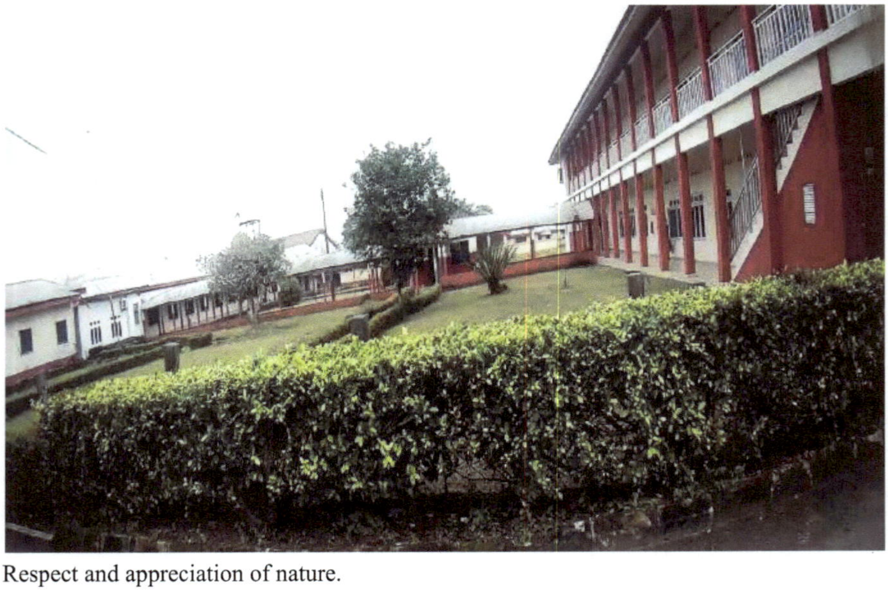

Fig. (6). Respect and appreciation of nature.

Although this photograph is a convincing representation of the respect and appreciation of nature, the author intends to also focus on the connection (*i.e.*, link) between the story building on the right and the bungalow on the left. Large hospitals that have many buildings must incorporate this feature into the construction within the premises of their hospitals. Uyo is in the South-South geopolitical zone of Nigeria and specifically in the Niger Delta Region. Rainfall is usually heavy and should not drench patients, patients' relatives, or employees during the process of transferring a patient from one part of the hospital to another part.

What the author desires to demonstrate from this photograph is the importance of government officials, agencies, and road construction companies paying attention to prevent disorderly driving in the vicinity of hospitals. Accidents have been known to occur right in front of hospitals because there was a failure to install the kind of impregnable concrete median in front of St. Luke's Hospital.

This photograph shows one of the features of many public buildings in Nigeria. There is the outdated belief that the public should have unrestrained access to a hospital. The author feels otherwise. Examples of security breaches taking place in hospitals in Nigeria have been reported in the news. This reality of insecurity should be considered a new normal in Nigeria, and our hospitals should not give every Tom, Dick, and Harry access as this may put patients and employees at risk. There is a "gatehouse" on the left but when this image was obtained, there was nobody to take control of the gate. Security personnel ought to open the gate to allow ingress and egress. The high metal structure in between the two buildings on the right is a stanchion to hold rigid plastic or metal plastic water tanks. Following the installation of the tank(s), water that is pumped into the tanks serves the buildings, which enjoy reticulation.

Unlike some properties in Nigeria that pay close attention only to the aesthetics of external walls and fences, the internal fence of St. Luke's Hospital receives equal attention as the external fences, as shown in Figs. (**1** and **7**).

This image is a further demonstration of the characteristic cleanliness and orderliness of St. Luke's Hospital, Anua Offot, Uyo, Akwa Ibom State.

This is another well-positioned ambulance. In another part of the hospital, just behind the ambulance, is another metal stanchion. There are three mounted black, durable plastic water tanks to serve the nearby hospital buildings. Another intended emphasis of this photograph is the guttering of the roof that enables the controlled dropping of water on the floor. This system protects the ground from "mini erosion" arising from a higher pressure if rainwater from the roof drops directly on the ground. It also protects the roof and walls of the building as it channels rainwater away from them. Pipework links the gutters with the ground.

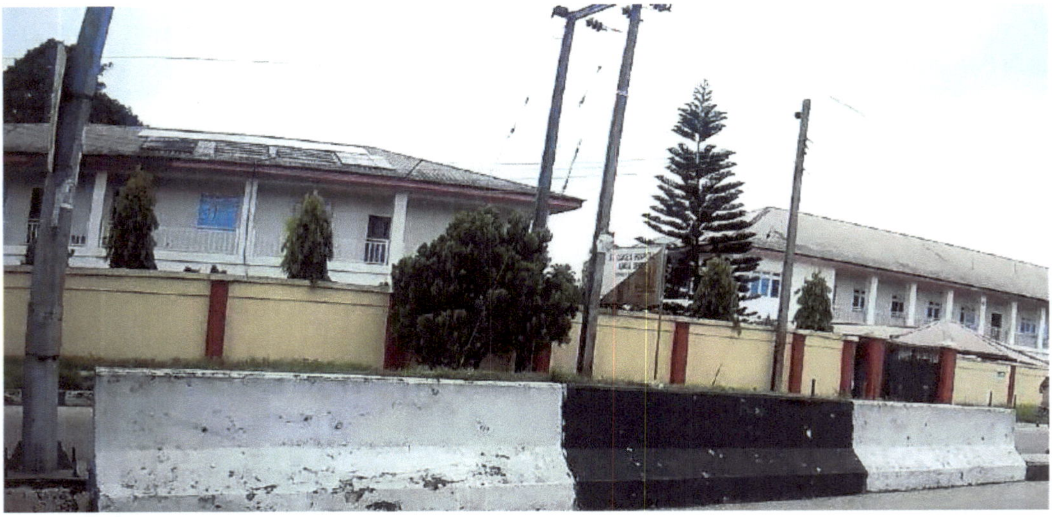

Fig. (7). Government's attention to road safety.

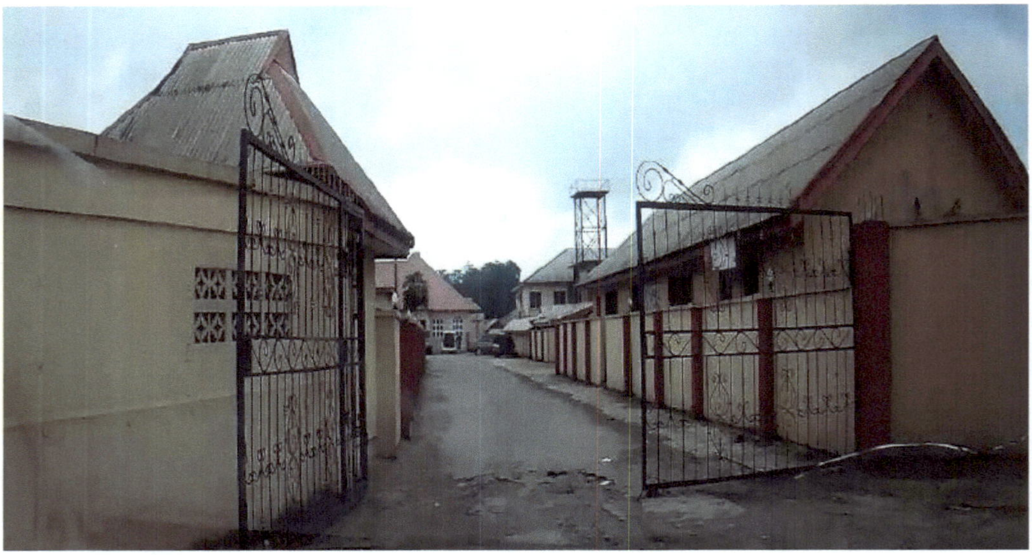

Fig. (8). Unrestrained access into a hospital.

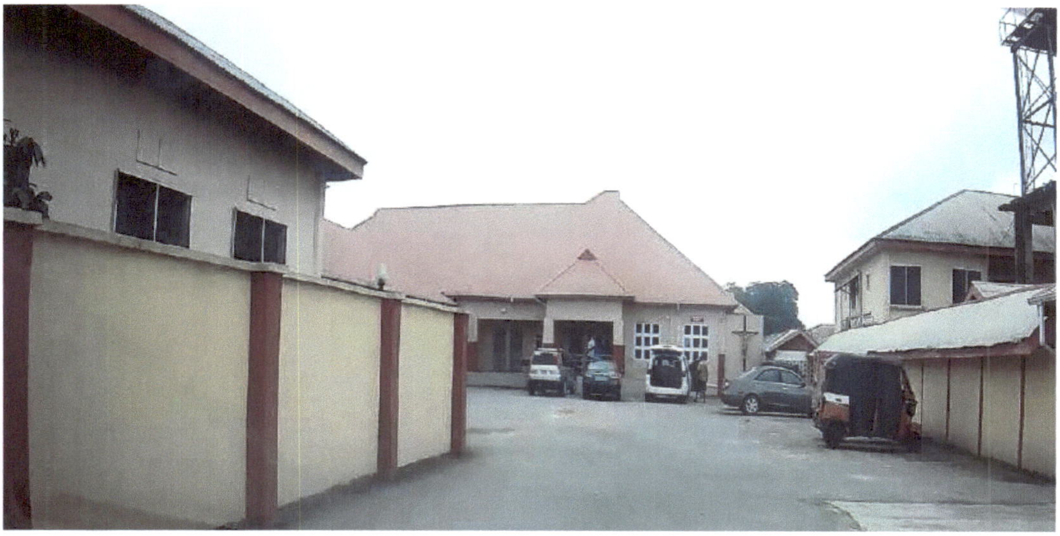

Fig. (9). The cleanliness and orderliness of St. Luke's Hospital.

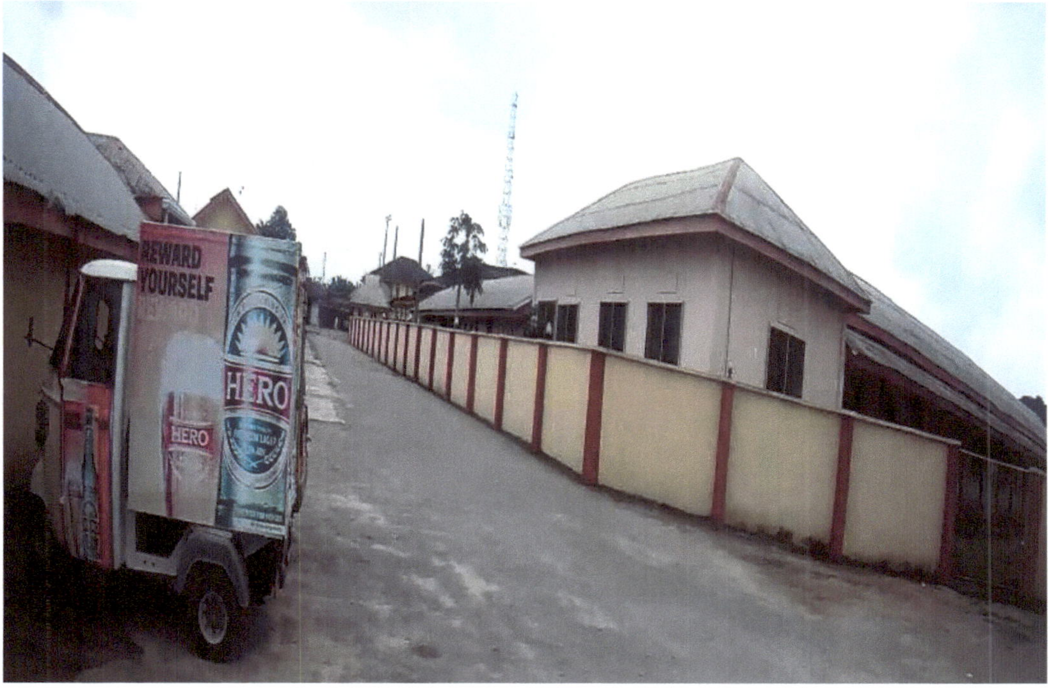

Fig. (10). Care for the internal fence of St. Luke's Hospital.

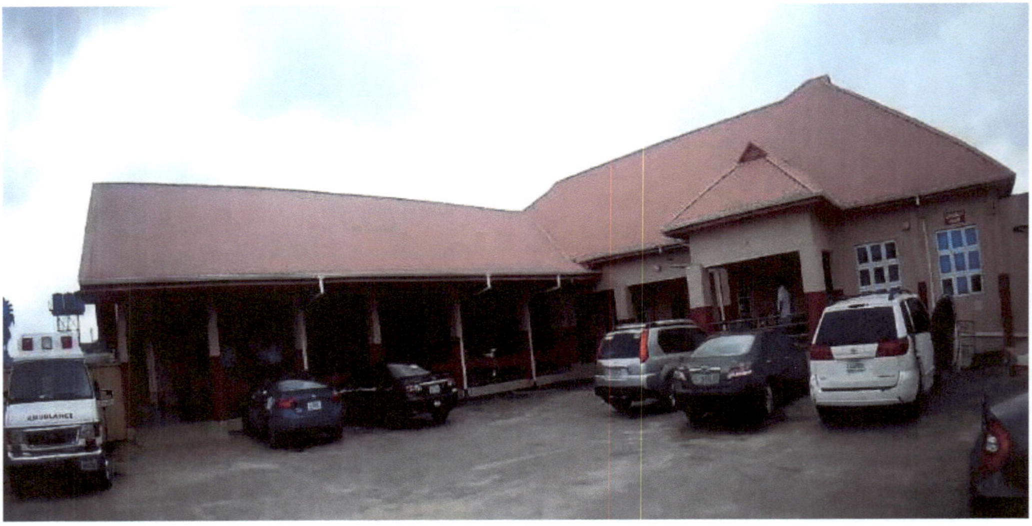

Fig. (11). Positioning of ambulances.

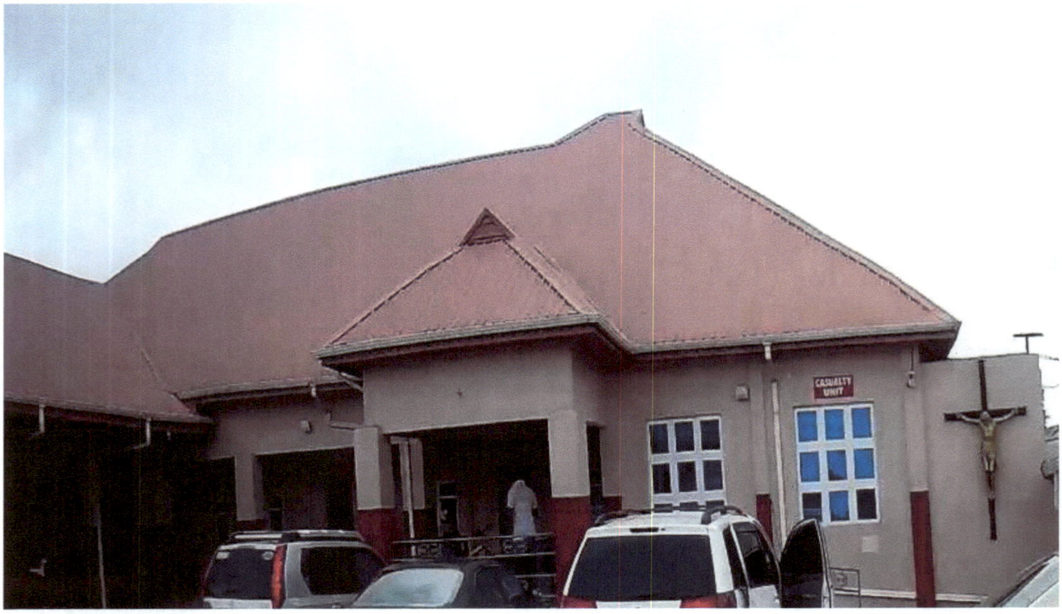

Fig. (12). This is the emergency unit.

Emergency units that are well planned and constructed are on the ground floor of a hospital with multiple floors or in a designated bungalow in the hospital's premises, as in St. Luke's Hospital, in which the unit goes by the name "Casualty Unit." To the right of the inconspicuous wall signage, "Casualty Unit," is a conspicuous sign of Jesus Christ's image on the Cross. Mission hospitals typically have one or more of such memorabilia. In this case, it shows that the owners of the hospital believe in power and depend on grace that is higher than their best human effort when rendering healthcare services, especially in critical cases.

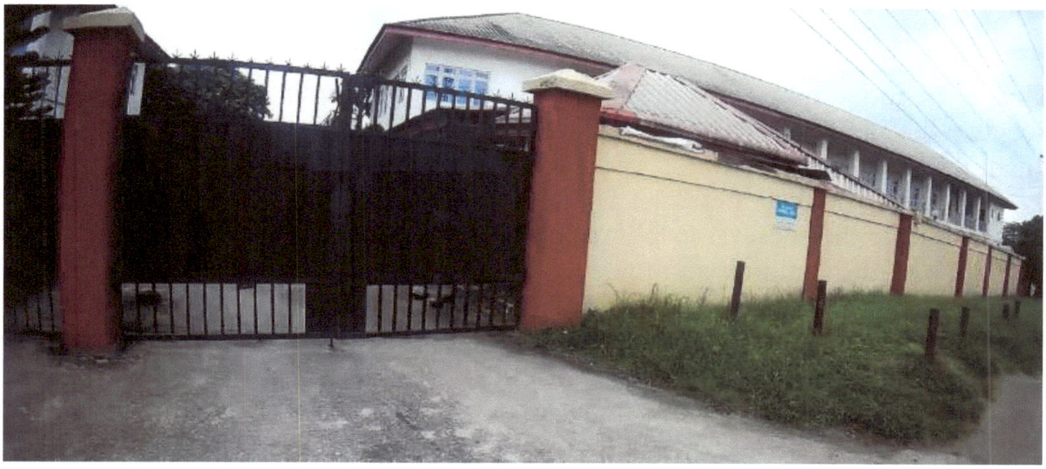

Fig. (13). Another gate.

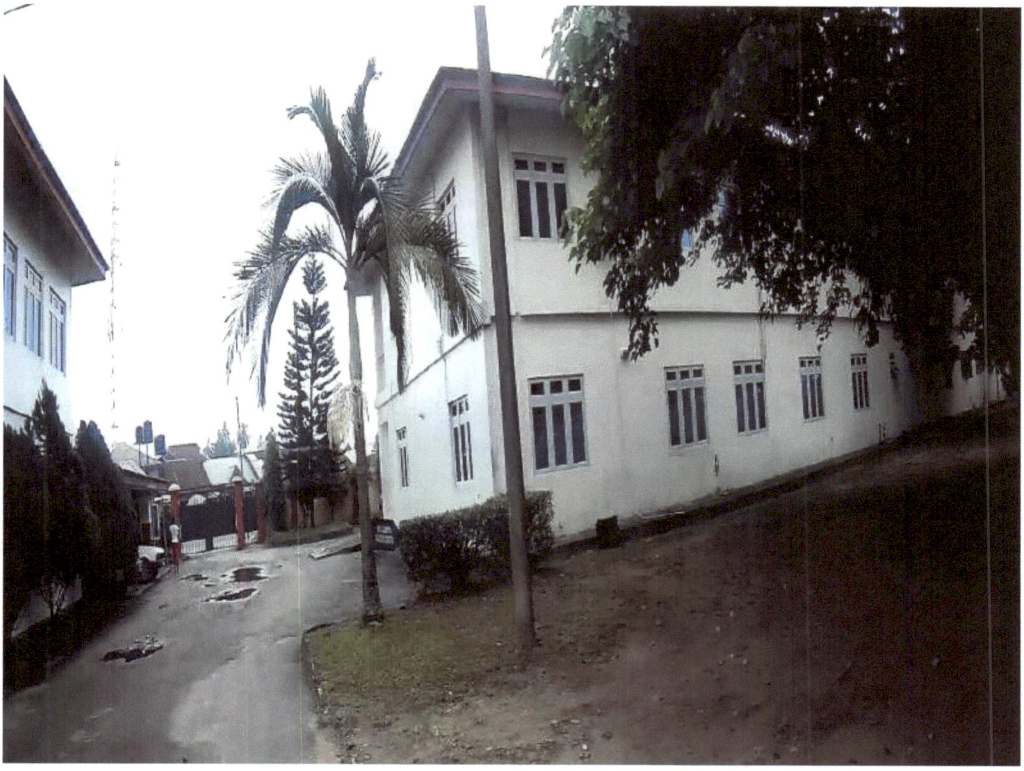

Fig. (14). The dialysis unit.

This photograph was taken at another gate of the hospital within minutes of one another. Gladly, this image is the opposite of (Fig. **8**) as it takes full account of security considerations. The black gate is in good aesthetic condition; the grass in front of the gate is equally so. The blue-and-white signage on the fence (to the right of the gate) states, "St. Luke's Hospital, Anua."

This last photograph shows the dialysis unit of the hospital on the right. This is because the photographer was making an exit from the hospital after capturing this image. The dialysis unit is located close to the gate. Referred patients brought by ambulance or their personal vehicles can readily identify this building and access it using the short ramp (shown on the right) at the front of the building. The ambiance of the building and the surroundings is reassuring. Despite the age of this significant hospital in Uyo, it is evident that the Catholic Diocese of Uyo had a vision and a solid plan for this facility, such that, by now, there would be no pressing need for satellite hospitals or clinics. Taking a futuristic view of some important hospitals is a sine qua non for success and maintenance of continuity. This Catholic hospital deserves a more detailed study and support from the Akwa Ibom State government, non-Catholics with means, in addition to devoted Catholic adherents.

(**N.B.:** This author declares that he is not a Catholic. This write-up on an exemplary long-term healthcare project is because it is noteworthy, worth emulating, and recommended by this author).

Management Housing Estate (MHE) Clinic, Eket; Qua Iboe Terminal (QIT) Clinic, Ibeno, and Bonny River Terminal (BRT) Clinic, Bonny Island, Nigeria

These clinics belong to and are operated by Mobil Producing Nigeria Unlimited (an arm of ExxonMobil in Nigeria) Seplat Energy Nigeria Ltd. The clinics are quintessential medical facilities. Ab initio, they are designed to render outpatient clinic services and occupational health services to registered clients. The main clinic of the three is registered to keep patients with emergency cases for not more than twenty-four hours, within which patients are discharged, or medical evacuation is activated to move the patient by land or by air to accredited private medical facilities with in-patient facilities, personnel, and services anywhere in Nigeria and sometimes outside Nigeria. The three clinics are in the Niger Delta Region of Nigeria. The facilities are well kept, and maintenance is at the forefront; every positive aspect that is mentioned in the earlier part of this chapter (and more) is observed in the three clinics. The clinics have always been linked by the most modern communication equipment available at any point in time, and these are upgraded as the clinics adjust their focus of services. One notable feature of this clinic group is that, despite not requiring physical expansion, it consistently delivers every medical service it intends to offer with excellence and reliability.

NNPC Medical Services Division (now NNPC Medical Services Limited)

The author of this work has spent a few years rendering services to the medical giant that belongs to Nigeria's oil company, the Nigerian National Petroleum Corporation (NNPC), which was recently renamed Nigerian National Petroleum Corporation Limited (NNPCL). This oil company in Nigeria operates the largest group of medical facilities among all oil companies in the country. Each of the hospitals is big. The facilities are well-kept. The equipment is top-notch and is regularly upgraded. From its time of transiting from rendering services only to employees, employees' qualified dependents, and retirees and their spouses to opening up its doors to the public and companies that register with their hospitals, things have improved. This is a hospital group that deserves a book to be written on it, and it is hoped that someone will take up this challenge to make widely known what this corporation and its medical facilities group have achieved over the years.

Eku Baptist Hospital, Eku, Delta State, Nigeria

This is the hospital where this author cut his teeth in medicine. It is where he was offered placement to spend the first year of his life as a doctor. This hospital was in existence for many years before 1981, when he had the wonderful opportunity of exposure to an American Surgeon (Dr. J. C. Abel), an American Obstetrician and Gynecologist (Dr. Martha Hagood), a Canadian Physician (Dr. Osborne), and an Indian Pediatrician. These core medical missionaries were of the Baptist Church background, and they made the hospital that was sited in a village between Sapele, Warri, Agbor, and Benin City a place that was functional and provided efficient medical services to patients beyond the then Bendel State (now Delta State and Edo State).

The functionality of this hospital had a lot to do with the commitment and sacrifice of the leadership mentioned above. There was also a Nigerian doctor among them, Dr. Agbowu. These all lived exemplary professional, private, and family lives. I still remember Dr. Martha Hagood consistently running what we, the young Nigerian doctors, considered an impossible schedule. This lady started her ward rounds at 06:00 hours and was usually there at 05:55 hours. How she maintained this specificity and regularity remains enigmatic to me (and, I believe, to any young doctor who passed through her extremely rigorous and disciplined tutelage). This author owes this highly esteemed specialist in Obstetrics and Gynecology, instilling in me a lasting aversion to lateness. However, he has yet to reach her high and unprecedented level.

The functionality of this hospital also depended on the following aspects:

- Ensuring that the hospital was in a self-sufficient status.
- Making accommodation available to all doctors and all senior doctors in the expansive hospital compound.
- Having a hostel for student nurses who were undergoing their registered nursing (RN) and registered midwifery (RM) programs within the hospital. They received unmatched training and always performed well. This incorporation of nursing training and internships for young, enthusiastic doctors provides the hospital with a continuous flow of disciplined doctors and nurses.
- Establishing residency in family medicine. Prior to this venture, first-year doctors always dealt with consultants directly, and this enabled them to hone their craft early and rapidly.
- This author remembers that he was very proficient in carrying out many procedures and gained operative skills in performing herniorrhaphy, cesarean section, and hemorrhoidectomy within the period of training and practice.
- Another way of ensuring functionality and efficient service delivery was getting supplies from the home missions in the United States and Canada; how they maintained the level of relationship was beyond our comprehension.
- Nigeria still suffers from the suboptimal electric power supply, but Eku Baptist Hospital has no such concerns; throughout the time the author of this work spent there, there was only a five-minute interruption of power supply, and Dr. J. C. Abell (who was not only a surgeon but also a pilot and an engineer) was instrumental to fixing it promptly.
- Maintenance of the green areas was a top priority and the entire hospital and staff quarters had regular water supply. The missionaries were futuristic in their planning and made sure they provided what they needed for their basic comfort, reliable and efficient medical services delivery, and maintenance of their facilities and equipment. This is replicable today but at a remarkably prohibitive cost.
- This hospital had a helicopter landing pad. Oil company patients with emergency cases used to be flown to this hospital, sited in a village, because of the assurance they had about receiving efficient healthcare services. This author, therefore, learned early that good services rendered in a village setting might be more valued by patients and corporate clients than poor services rendered in externally and aesthetically appealing medical facilities in cities.
- The last, though not the least, factor that this author remembers as being responsible for the functionality of this mission hospital and efficiency in the services it (and its personnel) provided consistently for decades was ensuring that the local workforce was on the same page with them. There was no insinuation or clear case of undermining the mission and vision of this hospital,

as the workers and community members saw the humility, simplicity, and integration of the White people (doctors) who did not look down on the Black people all around them. This suggests that for any medical facility to achieve its objectives, it must carry at least people in their neighborhood along and do everything to avoid antagonism.

The next set of hospitals that are described in this chapter includes two that are named, along with several others that remain unnamed. The account shall be brief for each, but only the last two shall have a pictorial representation of what applies to all of them, the positives and the negatives.

It is important to state that this short chapter attempts to condense the experience of hospitals that are in Nigeria. Some of the hospitals are in difficult terrain, while others are in enviable locations; some are five years old, while others have been in existence for about fifty years. The selection of the hospitals for inclusion in this chapter is to enable any prospective investor in the healthcare sector to gain from the positives and negatives by applying the practices of the former and avoiding the practices of the latter. It must also be stated that even abiding by the exemplary features of the contents of this chapter may not guarantee efficient service delivery; it may only attend to functionality in terms of the physical medical facility providing the human beings involved in the entire process the opportunity to utilize the building(s) and the physical attributes, including the installed and moveable equipment. So, the investor (government, organization, or private) should not scream "eureka" as this aspect of the hospital is akin to "the physical body" of a human being; we all know that "the body" in any morgue is bereft of "the soul and the spirit" and so is unresponsive to the passage of time in the morgue, meaning that the age of any lifeless object is immaterial as it is not subject to any activity on its own, not to mention efficiency that it may have experienced in the past or may have hoped or envisaged to experience but never did.

FullCare Hospital, Uyo, Akwa Ibom State

This is one of the private hospitals in Uyo. It is strategically located in the central part of the "original" Uyo. This expression was used because Uyo has developed to the extent that it is difficult to categorically state where its center is currently. However, it is close to the "town campus" of the University of Uyo, a Federal government-owned tertiary educational institution (the only one in Akwa Ibom State). The primary investor of this hospital is a professor of Family Medicine.

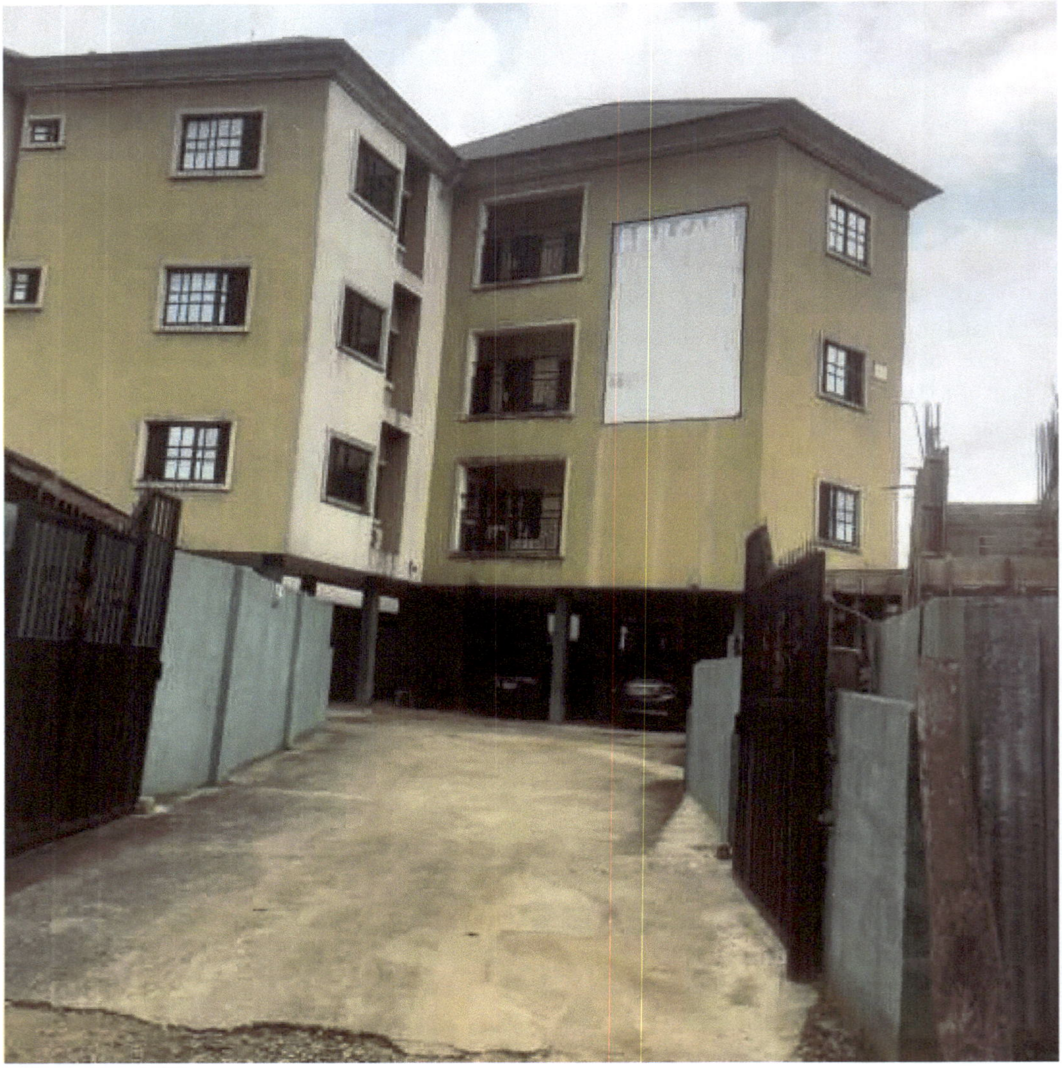

Fig. (15). A view of FullCare Hospital.

A view of FullCare Hospital, Uyo, facing the facility just before entering the open gates of the facility. This hospital is in a tight space with minimal grounds to space. However, to make room for parking and freedom of movement of patients, patients' relatives, and other clients like suppliers and maintenance personnel, the design and construction of this facility are ingenious. The ground floor is devoted to car parking, as illustrated. It gives the facility the semblance of having space. The next feature of this hospital is having multiple floors. Another feature is the name of the hospital – it is on the wall of the property. This signage is so conspicuous that it can be viewed and read from the nearby road. Although the inscription is not legible, it is the vertical image on the right side of the building; in height, it is approximately one-and-a-half floors high.

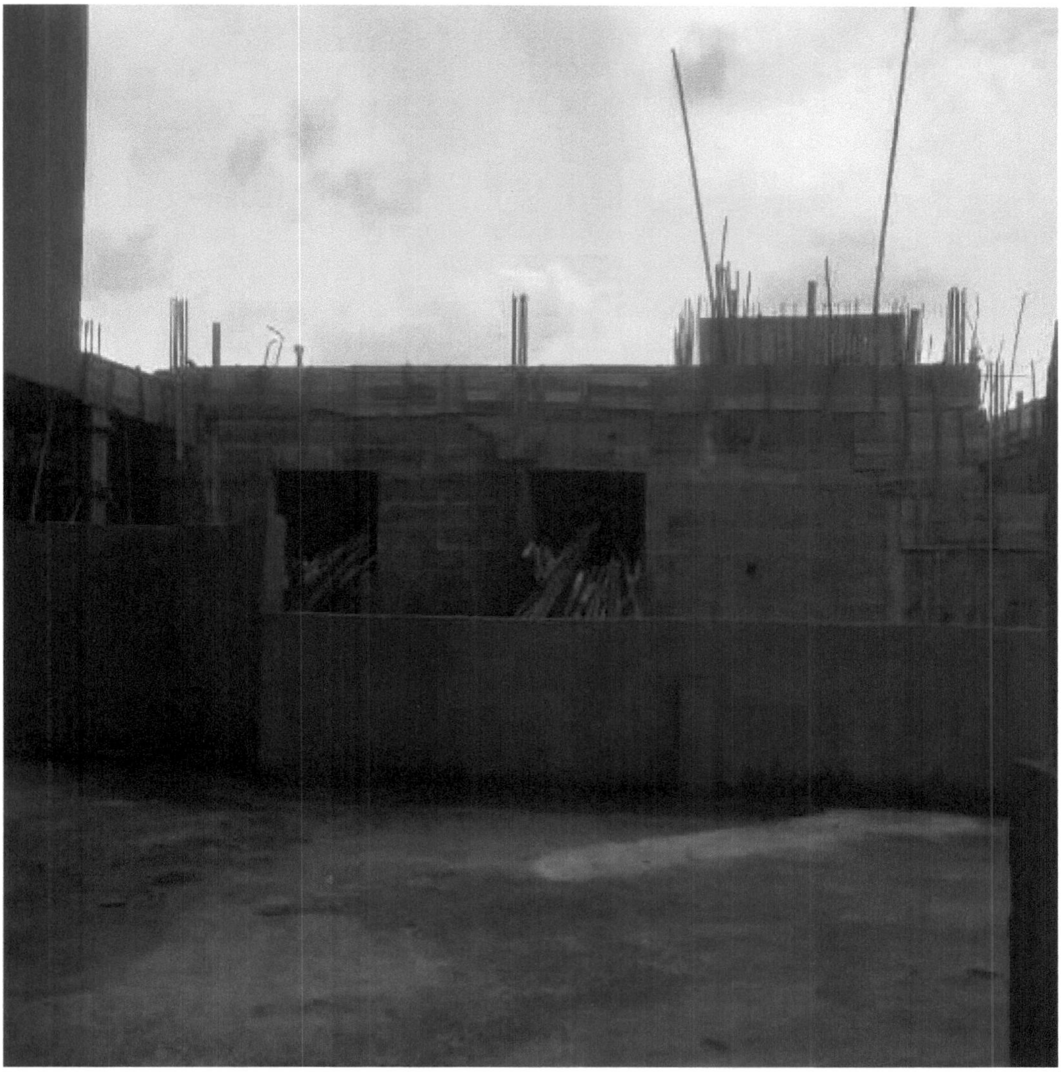

Fig. (16). The right side of the fence of the existing property.

This shows the right side of the fence of the existing property. It also shows a story building at the stage of decking; this decked property is outside the fence of the medical facility and, ordinarily, uncomfortably close to the hospital. On a close look at the left end of this image, there is another decked structure abutting the existing hospital.

The idea is that the property on one of the contiguous lands was available for sale, and the proprietors of FullCare Hospital, being apprised of this unexpected circumstance, did not give a second thought to doing everything possible to buy the property. The hitherto property was demolished, and approval was sought from the appropriate government authority to build a property to directly extend the existing hospital. With the authorization officially obtained, the building project commenced.

What strikes is that the owners of the hospital rightly chose not to pull down the fence that currently separates the two properties. They achieve privacy as the workers at the building construction site have no access to the hospital. The second benefit is the elimination or minimization of security risk if that fence was done away with, prematurely. The two properties shall be linked by pulling down the fence upon completion of the extension. This arrangement is better than having an annex in another location, no matter how close to the main hospital.

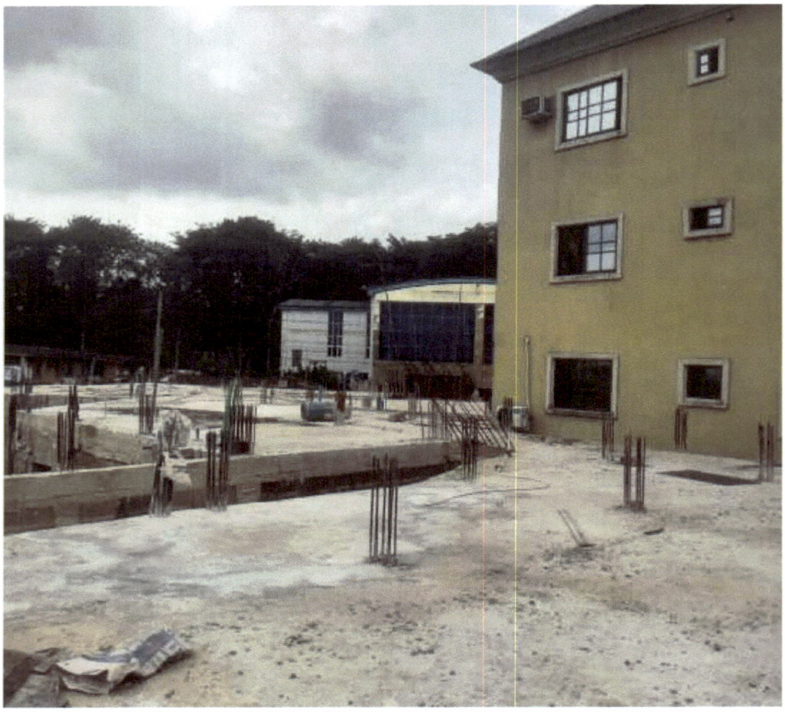

Fig. (17). The status of construction work.

This photograph shows the current status of construction work on the addition to FullCare Hospital, Uyo, Akwa Ibom State.

Three Hospital Stories in One

The next is a three-in-one story. This story comprises the observations of the author regarding three important hospitals. The hospitals are so important that they are not named and their locations shall not be mentioned other than that they are in Nigeria. They are as follows:

1. This hospital is in one of the cities of Nigeria. It started functioning barely twenty years ago. Within this period, the hospital has gained unprecedented patronage. It is located in a prominent part of the city, and there is accessibility as the road network is one of the best in the country. Currently, one of the nagging challenges of this hospital is the inadequacy of space. Space is insufficient within the fenced delineated property. There is also a shortfall in grounds outside the front buildings. The challenge is insoluble as more buildings are constructed in the limited space of this initially apparently wonderfully planned hospital; the compound looks and feels cramped. It is difficult for a new client to figure out where it is, whereas signage is inadequate. There are no earmarked muster points – at least, the author did not see anywhere they ought to be. The most frustrating challenge is parking. On busy days, vehicles are now parked on both sides of the road before and beyond the hospital. It takes an ill patient who needs to be directed by the driver fifteen minutes to find the only available parking space where the hospital's security personnel are. The patient walking an unduly long distance to get to the clinic is easily imagined. This hospital provides efficient services, but it is not possible to expand the land, although the available space is almost full of buildings now. The lesson here is not to underestimate a medical facility but to take a futuristic approach in the concept and planning of any hospital that is meant for a city that is known to (or is anticipated to) experience a high population growth rate.
2. The next hospital is also in Nigeria. In the case of this massive hospital, it was designed to render both service to the populace and training to prospective healthcare personnel. This hospital was allocated more than enough land, and despite being in existence for many years, it still has an ambiance that most hospitals in the city do not have and can only wish for. This hospital is about one hour from a major airport. Incidentally, it takes some people who live right in the city at the same time to get to this airport. Driving to this hospital is stress-free, but accessing the airport from the city could pose significant challenges especially at certain times of the day and depending on which part of the city one commences the journey to the airport.
3. The third hospital in this set is a private hospital. It is also in Nigeria. This hospital is in an enviable part of the city. This medical facility started on a

well-sited rented facility. The location of the rented property is so strategic that even when some young employees advised the proprietor and employer to buy the property, this advice was jettisoned. The employer eventually found the need to expand, but the original property had virtually become a "trademark." A contiguous property was erected, and the two buildings were linked. The lesson here is that it may occasionally be good to listen to and critically appraise the input of employees; this is because when employers treat employees as "stakeholders" and not dispensable and replaceable workers, the owners of a hospital business may obtain valuable advice gratis. There was dissatisfaction between the landlord of the original property and the proprietor of the top-notch medical facility. This author does not know the status of this hospital and whether the contending views of the principal actors have been resolved.

Cottage Hospital, Upenekang, Ibeno Local Government Area, Akwa Ibom State

There is a Cottage Hospital in Ibeno. It is strategically located in Upenekang along the Qua Iboe terminal road, as one approaches this massive on-shore terminal in one of the villages in Ibeno. Upenekang is the headquarters of Ibeno, which is one of the thirty-one local government areas in Akwa Ibom State. This state is in the Niger Delta Region of Nigeria; it owes its prominence to hosting Mobil Producing Nigeria Unlimited (part of ExxonMobil in Nigeria) in the State.

The Cottage Hospital, Ibeno, is a deep-seated desire of the traditional and political leaders of Ibeno and the entire community members to come true. The hospital is state government-owned. The hospital is less than twenty years old. It is designed and run as a secondary healthcare facility.

The following seven images present a pictorial description and assessment of this hospital, which was anticipated to play a crucial role for Ibeno and the surrounding communities. Although located in Ibeno, it serves not only local residents but also visitors and patients from neighboring states.

Figs. (**18** to **24**) are accompanied by brief comments regarding the condition of this facility as of the third quarter of 2024.

This photograph is of the Cottage Hospital, Ibeno, just before the fence and the gate. The fence and the gate are in dire need of painting. The gate is wide open. The gatehouse is not in proximity to the gate. The ground before the gate is concreted, while the ground from the gate towards the main hospital building is constructed with interlocking stones. Ingress and egress of anybody or group of people appear unrestricted.

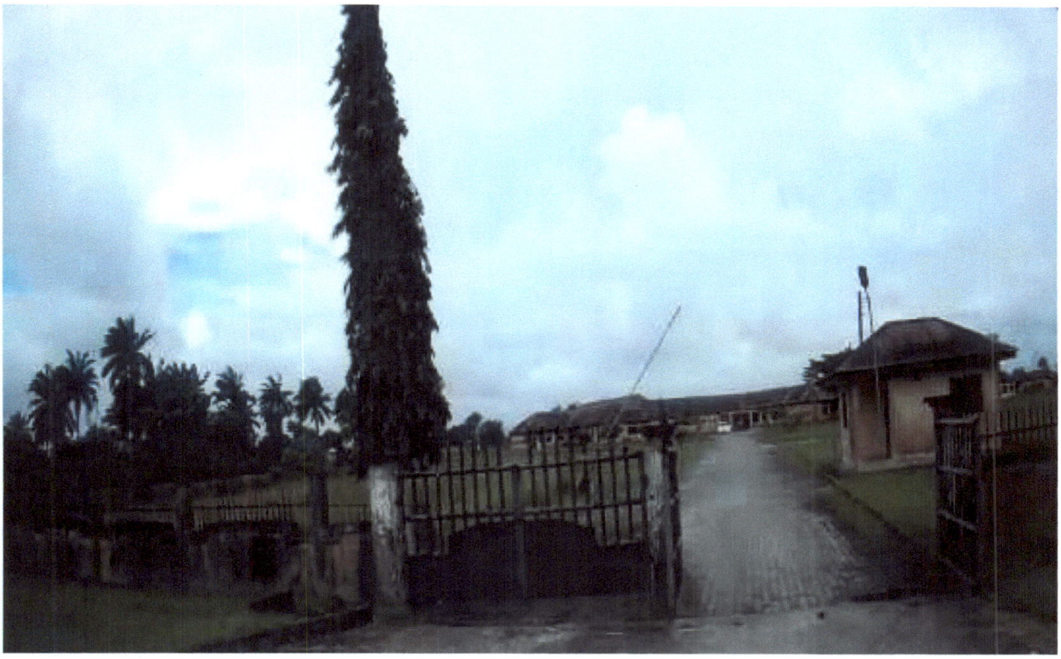

Fig. (18). The Cottage Hospital, Ibeno.

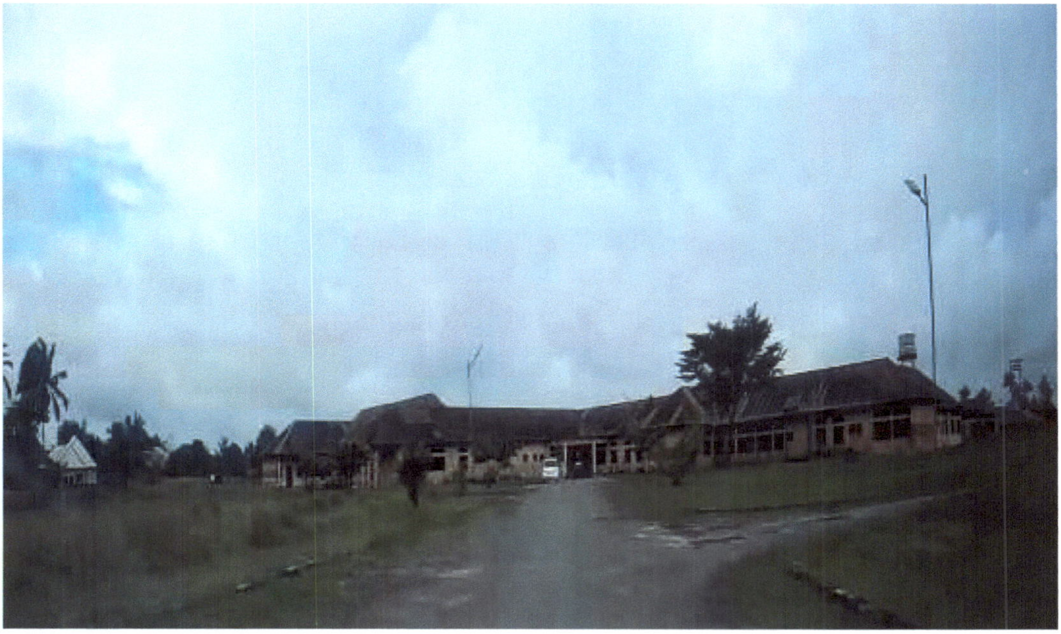

Fig. (19). Urgent need for maintenance.

This medical facility is rightly fenced around, but the fence (even the most visible part of it – the front) needs planned maintenance. Maintenance is what every non-building part of this massive compound begs for.

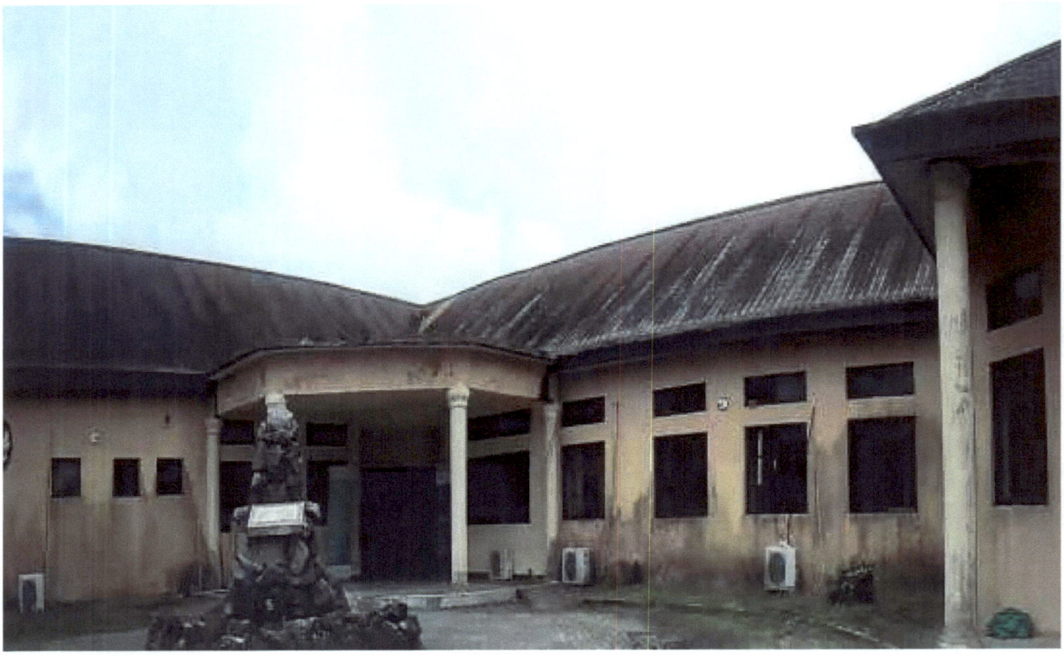

Fig. (20). The front of the main building.

Compared with many state government-owned and operated hospitals in this State, the Cottage Hospital at Upenekang, Ibeno, is a relatively new hospital. This photograph shows the front of the main building and a statue right in front of it. The roof, walls, and access road all need a good touch of maintenance work. With regard to the roof, there is no guttering, and adding guttering to this good structure would protect not only the roof but also the walls from rainwater.

A close view of the entrance to the main building of this hospital shows the concrete wall atop the concrete pillars exhibiting paint that has peeled off. The wall above the right inner pillar of this entrance is in bad shape, and leakage into it has led to the black discoloration seen in the photograph. The installation of guttering could have prevented this issue and should have been incorporated during the building's maintenance rather than simply scraping the wall and repainting it, as some contractors might do without proper supervision. This would help avoid a recurrence of the original construction flaw.

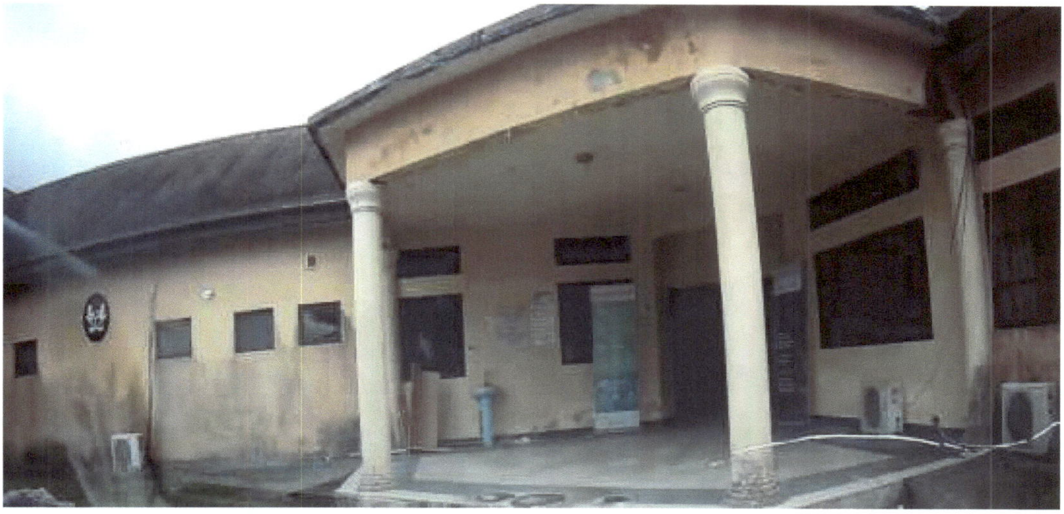

Fig. (21). A close-view photograph of the entrance to the main building.

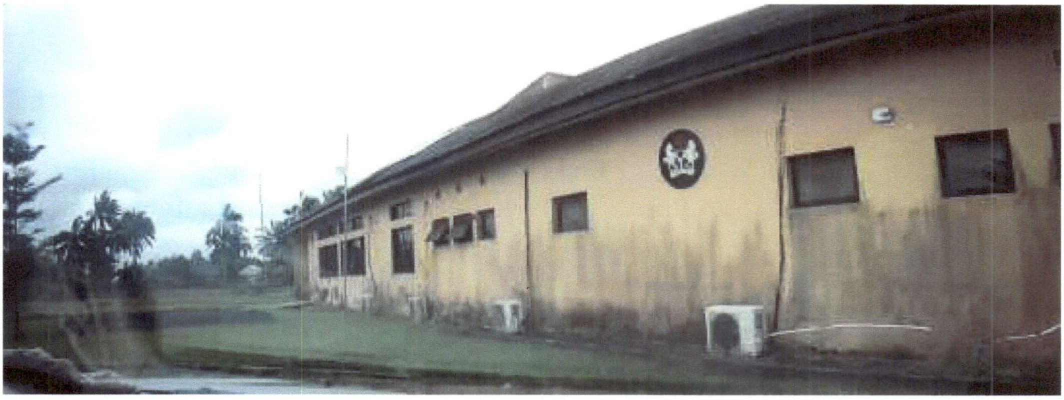

Fig. (22). Outdoor units of split-unit air conditioners.

This photograph is a part of the front building of this Cottage Hospital. It shows the outdoor units of split-unit air conditioners lying on bare ground. These components are much more expensive than the indoor unit that is inside the various parts of the hospital and needs no protection. These outdoor units are not protected in any form, although they are visible from the major road if a person is walking past and not inside a speeding vehicle driving past the hospital. Security and maintenance of government property are important. This is just an example of this twin challenge, which is found in many (if not all) the states in Nigeria. It is only when contractors do the right thing that there is hope of not purchasing equipment over and over again, depleting government funds for no cause.

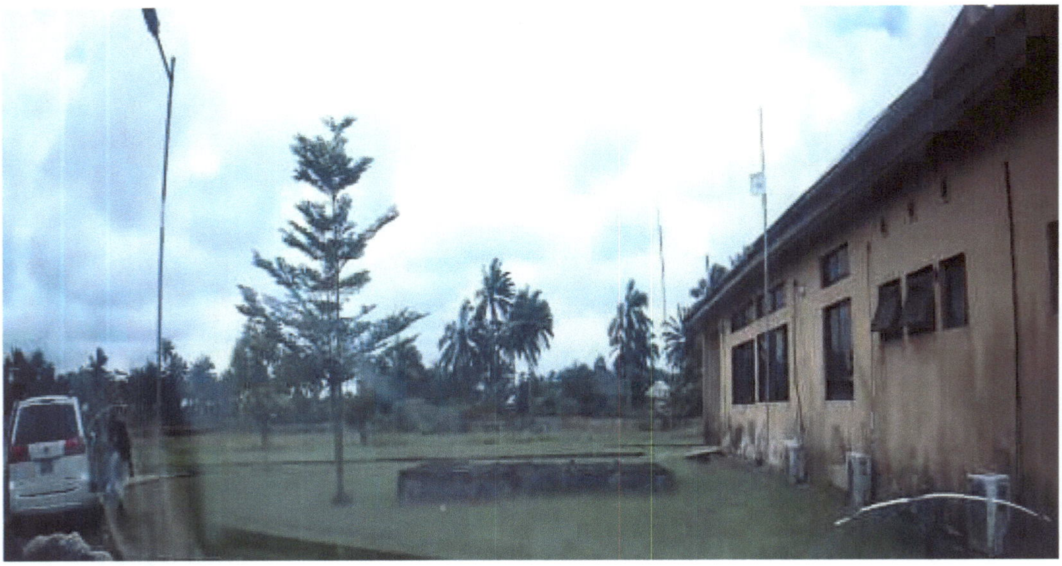

Fig. (23). The natural beauty of the compound.

This photograph, taken from the right side of the front of the medical facility, shows the natural beauty of the compound of this Cottage Hospital. It is clear that the state government had good intentions for this community, but something has obviously gone wrong. What is it? Only a detailed look at this medical facility by qualified professionals can unearth the challenges and proffer solutions to the government for the benefit of both the government and its citizens that the government intends to serve. The sooner the decay of this hospital is addressed, the better it will be for everyone in terms of reducing maintenance costs, achieving the hospital's intended functionality, and ensuring the efficient delivery of healthcare services to the intended beneficiaries.

Fig. (**24**) shows the Cottage Hospital, Upenekang, Ibeno Local Government Area in Akwa Ibom State as one approaches the gate. "Nature" across the Qua Iboe Terminal Road is natural and beautiful. "Nature" within the compound of this secondary care medical facility should be properly maintained—sooner rather than later.

CONCLUSION

Functionality of every component of the physical aspect of a hospital of any size is imperative if the personnel who render healthcare services within that facility will do it successfully and efficiently. It is conceded that there are other factors, such as conditions of services, level of teamwork among the employees, degree of discipline, and leadership by example, but even when all these factors are perfect, the employees need a "body" within which to function and convince their patients that they are doing it efficiently. That body is the "medical facility," including its immediate environment.

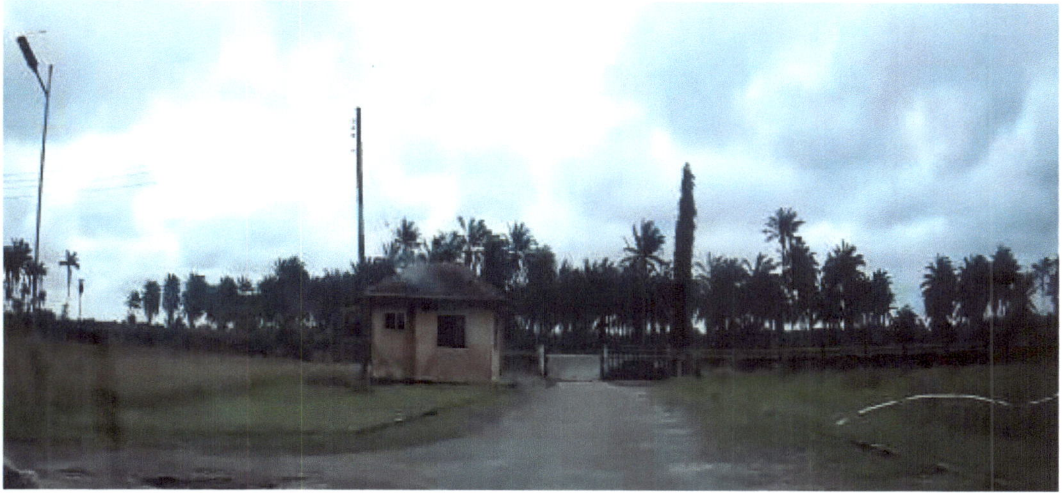

Fig. (24). Approaching the hospital gate.

REFERENCES

[1] Planning. Business Jargons. Available from: https://businessjargons.com/planning.html

[2] McCabe JD. Analogy to a building design. Network Analysis, Architecture, and Design 2007; 3. Available from: https://www.sciencedirect.com/topics/engineering/building-design

[3] Schoenmaker D, Strumeyer M, Strange T. Unique challenges of hospital construction. Hospital Construction: A Guide to Design & Construction of Healthcare Facilities. ProCore Solutions 2024. Available from: https://www.procore.com/library/hospital-construction

[4] USAID . Primary health care project. standard operation procedure for facility and equipment maintenance management in primary health care clinics iraq. 2013. Available from: https://pdf.usaid.gov/pdf_docs/PA00KD86.pdf

[5] Ebekozien A, Duru OSD, Dako OE. Maintenance of public hospital buildings in Nigeria – an assessment of current practices and policy options. Journal of Facilities Management. Emerald Insight 2022. Available from: https://www.emerald.com/insight/content/doi/10.1108/JFM-11-20-0-0088/full/html?skipTracking=true [http://dx.doi.org/10.1108/JFM-11-2020-0088]

[6] Zanna UA. Abandoned public hospitals pushing nigerian villages into deadly health crisis. HumAngle 2024. Available from: https://humanglemedia.com/abandoned-public-hospitals-pushing-nigerian-villages-into-deadly-health-crisis/

[7] Sabiu M. Gov sani laments abandonment of 32 general hospitals in kaduna. Latest News – Nigerian Tribune 2024. Available from: https://tribuneonlineng.com/gov-sani-laments-abandonment-of-32-general-hospitals-in-kaduna/

[8] Akinlotan O. Inside abandoned 250-bed ogun hospital where termites, others are patients. Punch 2024. Available from: https://punchng.com/inside-abandoned-250-bed-ogun-hospital-where-termites-others-are-patients/

[9] Kapologwe NA, Meara JG, Kengia JT. Development and upgrading of public primary healthcare

facilities with essential surgical services infrastructure: a strategy towards achieving universal health coverage in Tanzania. BMC Health Serv Res 2020; 20: 218. [http://dx.doi.org/10.1186/s12913-020-5057-2] [PMID: 32183797] [PMCID: PMC7076948]

[10] Warda L. Is your hospital safe for children? Applying home safety principles to the hospital setting. Paediatr Child Health 2004; 9(5): 331-4. Available from: https://pubmed.ncbi.nlm.nih.gov/19657520/ [PMID: 19657520] [PMCID: PMC2721182]

[11] Chaff LF. Safety in health care facilities. J Healthc Prot Manag 1991; 8(1): 1-22. Available from: https://pubmed.ncbi.nlm.nih.gov/10116979/ [PMID: 10116979]

[12] Top 10 security challenges facing hospitals and how to solve them. Accutech Healthcare Security Solutions 2024. Available from: https://www.accutechsecurity.com/top-10-security-challenges-facing-hospitals-and-how-to-solve-them/

CHAPTER 5

Getting the Best Out of Hospital Employees

Inyang Ukot[1,*]

[1] *RST Clinics Ltd., Federal Housing Estate, Uyo, Akwa Ibom State, Nigeria*

Abstract: The idea behind this Chapter, "Getting the best out of hospital employees," is the reality that there are many hospitals in Nigeria that do not lack patients, but what they lack are hospital employees who, for one reason or another, do not or cannot give the best to their employers or patients. When and where this happens, the physical edifice of the affected government hospitals and the smaller facilities owned by individuals and organizations exist mainly to pay salaries and to "stay open" to the public. The clientele dwindles over time and such medical facilities become abandoned where the negative and unprogressive trend is not stemmed. Since it is difficult to repurpose a purpose-built hospital, particularly large hospitals (government or private) become liabilities rather than the assets they were intended to be. This scenario is presented first with the purpose being to discourage any employer or investor from allowing this to happen to them, their business, or social services project. Unquestionably, the best asset that any hospital has is the human resources. How to get the best out of hospital employees is consequently the best objective of any hospital, its management officials, and owners/proprietors.

Interestingly and almost peculiarly, a reasonably large hospital in Nigeria, in addition has features of a hotel, restaurant, bank, typical office or institution, school, land transportation outfit, and more. Hospital employees or personnel are, therefore, not only the core healthcare professionals like doctors, nurses, pharmacists, laboratory scientists, and medical records personnel but also administrative personnel, lecturers, teachers, security personnel, cooks and restauranters, janitorial staff members, employees of banks that have outlets in the hospital premises, drivers, and more. Sadly, carrying along sixty percent of these personnel does not give the institution a pass mark in the minds, eyes, words, and social medial postings of patients and their family members. This is because a patient may feel impressed right from the hospital's entry and exit gates just because of the treatment that they receive the first time or every time they have cause to go to the hospital. On the other hand, they may become disgruntled at the point of entering the compound of the hospital or anywhere in between there and their leaving the hospital – and this could be the handiwork of one hospital personnel or more than one such employee. Despite the training that hospital employees (core personnel or support staff members) receive during training in their various schools, their attitude towards clients and the level of service they render are generally based on the individual. This chapter is to show that it ought not to be so; it should be institution-

* **Corresponding author Inyang Ukot:** RST Clinics Ltd., Federal Housing Estate, Uyo, Akwa Ibom State, Nigeria; E-mail: inyang.ukot@yahoo.com

Impact Clinics Ltd. has since replaced the former company name RST Clinics Ltd.

alized. Every hospital must establish the standards on which it wants its employees to function and, at the same time, know and remember that the treatment it gives to its employees goes a long way to determining what services it can extract from these employees. The immediately preceding sentence simply means that if employees' salaries are withheld for months, indiscipline is condoned, time for work is flouted with no consequences, leaders fail to show good examples, there is harassment in the workplace, fairness in handling personnel matters becomes an unnoticed or irrelevant "man overboard," there is lack of training and employees' progression in the workplace is irrational or inexplicable, or retired employees are not paid their benefits for months or years, it becomes very difficult to obtain from employees that commitment to work that is integral in rendering excellent services naturally.

Keywords: Accreditation process, ACLS, Advanced cardiac life support, Advanced practice roles, Advanced technological devices, Advanced trauma life support, American hospital association, ATLS, Attitude, Basic life support, BLS, Burnout, CGFNS, Client services, Clinical training exposes, Conditions of service, Developed countries, Developing countries, Emigration, Emotional support, Greener pastures, Health risk assessment, Inconducive work environment, Interactive case studies, Levels of equipment, National council licensure examination, NCLEX, Nursing and midwifery council of nigeria, PALS, Pediatric advanced life support, Personnel, Professional development, Retired nurses, Retirements and succession, Retiring nurses, Rural areas, Simulation, Shift work, Standardized documentation, Standardized nursing care, Task trainers, Training, Training, Virtual clinical tools, Young nurses.

INTRODUCTION

This chapter is on hospital employees; these consist of at least four groups, *viz.*: medical professionals, other healthcare professionals, administrative professionals, and support members of staff. Writing on every professional in these groups would take an entire book. This chapter does not attempt to start what it cannot achieve, and so its author has chosen to use the most ubiquitous personnel (in the sense that wherever they are not present, the facility may not be rightly designated as a medical facility). In the healthcare industry, the progress and impact made by the various professionals depend partly on the level and efficiency of the training that the future professionals receive in their years in school and the formative years during practice. The challenge of achieving and sustaining this ideal is immense. In advanced countries where training and practice are well structured and highly regulated, it is still a challenge; in developing countries where the struggle is multifaceted, the development of the healthcare sector and its professionals is a monumental challenge. These personnel are nursing personnel, and the reader should bear with the author in using them to represent every other personnel found in a typical hospital.

Training and Practice in the Nursing Profession

In the USA, for example, the American Association of Colleges of Nursing (AACN), in its 2024 fact sheet on salaries and instructional and administrative nursing faculty, documents that the mean ages of doctoral-prepared faculty at the highest levels ranged between 49.6 and 61.2 years; the age bracket was lower for nurse faculty with master's degree [1]. This shows that there is a shortage even in the USA. The healthcare burden is higher in developing countries, and very few have personnel at this elevated level to train nurse faculty who would engage in the training of nursing personnel at lower levels. Until the relevant authorities find and implement a solution for this challenge of teaching professionals shortage, the hope of achieving top-notch nursing services consistently and globally could prove to be a mirage. The challenge is even direr in developing countries. It is natural for employees to age, but this inevitably shortens the number of productive years available for nurses and other healthcare educators to teach and mentor the next generation. In Nigeria, for example, some accredited centers for training nurses are inundated with nursing students, and this could wear out the lecturers.

Regarding retirements and succession of nursing faculty between 2016 and 2025, this work by Fang and Kesten suggested that there is an impending departure by the retirement of about 33% of top nursing faculty that were in service in 2015 [2]. This would not only negatively impact the training of high-level personnel to teach upcoming nursing postgraduate and undergraduate students but could also threaten the future nursing workforce. As mentioned in the previous paragraph, any negative impact on healthcare professionals' training and practice in advanced countries tends to reflect a greater (and unreported or underreported) negative impact in developing countries. Unfortunately, in developing countries, the conditions of service are far from satisfactory, and when given the opportunity, these high-level academics would rather leave their countries for "greener pastures" or take up political appointments that offer higher remunerations and added perks of high office, these could permanently prevent them from returning to the "classrooms or lecture halls" after their tenure.

A further challenge is the remuneration imbalance between high-level nursing practitioners and high-level teaching professionals in nursing. While the median salary of nurse practitioners, nurse anesthetists, and nurse midwives in 2023 was $129,480 (and the hourly pay was $62.25), the pay of a professor for the corresponding period was less by about $36,000 (at $ 93,958) [3, 4].

At the time of the research by Anarado, Agu, and Nwonu that led to their publication in 2016, the results of the study that took place in the South-Eastern zone of Nigeria revealed findings which included the following hindrances: teachers not participating in supervision of students, students proceeding to gain clinical experience without ensuring that they satisfied the requirement of completing academic and non-clinical (patient-based) practical work, constraints in opportunities for students in the degree program to return for supervised demonstrations and independent laboratory performance. The students in the diploma program did not have an optimal number of teachers, nor did they enjoy the adequacy of clinical instructors or patient numbers to meet the requirements of their training [5]. These findings ought to be retested nearly ten years later to determine if these gaps have been closed or if they are wider.

The study by Aghedo *et al.* on the experiences of graduate nursing respondents who communicated with the Nursing and Midwifery Council of Nigeria included the following findings: the most common means of communication were telephone and email. Accessibility to those who desired to make physical visits to the Council's zonal offices was a challenge. Although communication by electronic means was preferable, the Council's system was not satisfactorily interactive. The low level of active involvement of Council personnel in resolving the challenges of professions dents the image of the regulatory body [6]. Although this council may have good intentions, it, like many public institutions in Nigeria (and possibly in other developing countries), should be continuously given attention to ensure upgrades to meet the expectations of the Council and the professionals they are meant to serve. In this way nurses will have a positive and pleasant connection with their regulatory body and allow that connection to percolate to their patients everywhere they are in the country.

From the findings of the research published as "Making Nurses and Nursing Care Visible in Nigeria. A Review of Standardized Nursing Care" Ojo *et al.* recommended, among other things, that "There is a dire need to inculcate standardized nursing languages into the curriculum of undergraduate in all the schools in the geopolitical zones at the Baccalaureate and graduate levels in Nigeria." [7] From doing this, it will be possible, over time, for the nursing language to trickle down and reflect in the practice of nurses nationally. The six geopolitical zones serve as major reference points for governance in Nigeria, and implementing this initiative at that level would help ensure that every nurse and the patients they care for benefit from this advancement, which has already become standard in many developing countries.

In a study conducted at an institution in Ogun State, Nigeria, the activities of nurses did not have adequate incorporation and utilization of nursing processes. The authors recommended a mandate of supervision and inclusion of the nursing process in continuing professional education of nursing personnel. This would help to improve the services that nurses render in Nigeria and other developing countries, especially if patients in the numerous peripheral hospitals in this highly populated African country feel the benefit of implementing the desirable mandate [8].

Perhaps because the nursing practice regulatory body has not mandated the application of standard nursing language using the standardized nursing care plan (SNCP), its use in the country's hospitals is selective so far [9 - 11]. Even where standardized nursing care plans have been implemented it is difficult to put them into practice optimally due to inconducive work environment, suboptimal levels of equipment, training, personnel, and attitude [12, 13]. Achieving success in the matter of standardized documentation of nursing practice would significantly improve the service that nurses render to patients and positively impact the practice of other practitioners like doctors and pharmacists.

For improvements in the current unsatisfactory status of services that every healthcare profession renders to patients to take place, be maintained, and extend to advancements in each of the professions in this sector, there must be a revamp in everyone's attitude, determination, focus on excellence in services delivery and empowerment by government, representatives of the various classes of ownership of medical facilities, and fairness in the treatment that employers give to their employees, and the employees give to their employers and patients.

Much of the rest of this chapter describes the training and practice of nursing professionals in Nigeria and compares it with nursing in advanced countries using the United States of America as a template. It briefly touches on the differences and peculiarities of nursing training and practice in these countries; it also examines the challenges that each practice setting encounters regarding nursing personnel staffing levels. In Nigeria, nursing students undergo didactic and clinical training. The didactic aspect of their training consists of structured lectures and practical work. Clinical training exposes them to patients and other professionals with whom nurses interact. When they complete their training, nursing students sit for the professional exams, which are held four times a year. When they succeed, they are employed in an arm of the workforce. This may be at the federal level, state level, or local government level if they choose to join public service; it could also be in the private healthcare sector. There are other opportunities, as documented in the rest of this book. The United States of America (USA) requires every nursing student to sit and pass the National Council Licensure Examination (NCLEX), irrespective of where they were trained in the USA or Canada. Nurses who trained outside these two countries are required to have at least two years of practice experience as nurses before they qualify to sit for an NCLEX examination. The examination may be written in selected centers in designated countries like Nigeria, Ghana, India, and Pakistan. These countries' nationals make up a reasonable bulk of foreign-trained nurses who are already working in the USA. The NCLEX is a multiple-choice exam that tests a student nurse's critical thinking. The examination may be for registered nurses, NCLEX-RN, or for practical nurses, NCLEX-PN. Foreign nurses are required to obtain certification from the Commission on Graduates of Foreign Nursing Schools (CGFNS) international. The CGFNS Certification Program® is meant for nurses who wish to work as nurses in the United States but were trained outside the USA. Those who are admitted to the program are registered nurses (RN), as they are considered first-level general nurses [14]. CGFNS is the world's largest organization set up for the evaluation of nursing and allied health profession credentials.

Nurses constitute the largest segment of professionals among all healthcare professions worldwide. Nurses are active participants in rendering efficient team-based services. The training and professional development of nurses enable them to play their role satisfactorily. Therefore, a well-trained workforce is the key to high-quality staff and properly functioning departments and hospitals. Like for other personnel who work in the hospital environment, training is an important foundational aspect of the lifelong learning experience. It is very difficult to build on poor or sub-standard training. Good quality training, on the other hand, is a good starting point. The training of nurses or any group of healthcare professionals rests on institutions, facilities, curriculum, time, and prospects for the professional within a country or globally. Professional development is subsumed in training for the purpose of this write-up.

According to the Nursing and Midwifery Council of Nigeria (NMCN), Nigeria also has two entry-level programs, registered general nurse (RN) and registered midwife (RM). In both the USA and Nigeria, each student must successfully complete an approved nursing program and must pass the licensing exams in the United States. Success at the NCLEX leads to receiving a license to practice nursing either as a registered nurse (RN) or a practical nurse (PN). In Nigeria, a pass at the NMCN exams licenses the candidate to practice as a registered general nurse [RN] or a registered midwife [RM]). In the USA, many nurses go further and specialize at the master's or doctorate levels; the same applies to Nigerian-trained nurses, though the higher-level academic nurses are fewer. Over the years, the numbers have increased as many young people have become aware of the potential opportunities that are available for nurses.

In Nigeria, nurses have the basic qualification in general nursing (RN). Most nurses who desire to have additional qualifications opt for midwifery, and so they become registered midwives (RM). In Nigeria, the Registered Midwife (RM) qualification is highly valued, and many Registered Nurses (RNs) feel incomplete without it, leading most nurses to obtain both RN and RM credentials. Some nursing students, however, enroll directly in the Bachelor of Science (BSc) program in Nursing Science, through which they acquire these qualifications as part of the curriculum, along with a first degree.

The trainee (prospective nurse or graduate nurse) should have made a solid and well-informed decision or choice to become a nurse and remain one. A number of factors may be responsible for a person choosing to become a nurse, and while some are good, like a deep-seated desire to render humane care for the ill and infirm and the desire to advance the nobility of the profession, other reasons may be frivolous like assessing nursing as a simpler course; recommendation of the course by parents, relations or friends; search for a means of earning income and a means of livelihood; captivation with nurses' uniforms (which are getting more and more attractive with time).

Trainers of nurses have the potential to make or mar nursing trainees, so it is important for the nursing profession to ensure that their academic staff and those who groom nursing students in their months or years of practical exposure know that their work could leave positive or negative, but indelible, marks or impression on the budding nurses. Young nurses copy their seniors, and what they end up giving out in the future in terms of service could well reflect what they got from their trainers. Good services, therefore, are expected from people who are well trained. Trainers may be academic or practical personnel; exposure is usually to the academic personnel (nurse educators) first and later to the practitioners.

Managers of nurses' training may not be the ones who train nurses directly, but people who design the curriculum of nursing training and handle the examination and certification processes. They are also the ones who supervise continuing nursing education programs.

The content of the nursing curriculum must meet both the academic needs and practical requirements of current nursing practice globally and nationally. The summary is that the standardization in content and delivery of nursing training should ensure that when a nurse receives qualification, the minimum expectation should be readily demonstrated by a registered nurse (RN) or a registered midwife (RM), irrespective of where the nurse received training. The same applies to students who obtain a bachelor's degree in nursing.

Institutions of nursing provide the environment for training. They could be new, old, or somewhere in between in terms of age. In Nigeria, some of the old institutions, especially the ones owned by or associated with mission hospitals, were frequently located close to their mission facilities (administrative, hospital, or residential). Some are in what have now become cities, while others are still in rural or semi-urban areas. Institutions owned by the government are usually in more accessible places. The availability of utilities at some locations has a way of attracting a variety of people, including nurses, especially if there are also training centers for the nursing profession. The utilities and services include water, electricity, and other things that make life easier and more comfortable, like the Internet, a relatively good quality road network, reasonable means of transportation, good and affordable accommodation, supermarkets, shopping malls, places of worship, and schools. More specifically, institutions for training nurses (the majority of the students being females) should provide them with at least basic comfort as this affects the trainees' psyche positively. The same thing happens if the health institutions they are posted to for practical experience maintain expected standards.

In the USA, there are public, private, and military training institutions that offer nursing training. Every training institution obtains accreditation at the state level. Each state in the USA not only uses general criteria as a baseline but also ensures that the graduates of nursing schools would not fail to meet preset standards for the practice of nursing in their state. Institutions used as training centers should be well selected and undergo regular and thorough accreditation exercises. The purpose is to ensure that professional training facilities and general facilities are well maintained and are at par with determined standards. This means that the expected range and functionality of training materials/equipment are in every training center. It does prospective nurses and the nursing profession no good if such centers lack qualified academic personnel and other members of staff do not have some essential training equipment or the ones they used to have are beyond repairs or have outlived their usefulness. In the USA, healthcare facilities counter shortages by implementing "float pools." "Float pools" are a list of available nursing staff that can be deployed from one unit or center to another.

Time is of the essence in the training of nurses. Everyone involved in training must make optimal use of time. Students must attend lectures and not skip practical sessions; trainers must be punctual and spend the entire teaching period teaching and supervising students; at other times, the curriculum may indicate when to demonstrate procedures to their students. They should also ensure that they spend the time allotted for other things judiciously. Missing out on training in some fundamental areas or topics may create deficiencies in nurses; it should not be surprising that nursing students who had such experiences may not give their best to their employers and patients in the future.

Expectedly, the scope of nursing practice is very broad and tends to mimic the specialties in the field of medicine. The practice of nursing has a lot to do with the level of care a particular health institution offers to its clients and requires the services of nurses. The institutions may provide primary health services, secondary health services, or tertiary health services. In the Nigerian setting, primary health services are provided in health clinics, health posts, health centers, and comprehensive health centers. Secondary health services are usually provided in general hospitals and cottage hospitals. Teaching hospitals and some specialist hospitals operated by federal government or state governments render tertiary health care services to patients. Apart from these public institutions, there are private hospitals of various sizes that provide secondary and tertiary health care. In Nigeria and other developing countries, there are also health institutions that nurses can operate on their own with the proviso that they do prompt referral of patients with cases beyond the scope of the approved health facility, like a maternity home.

Nurses are engaged in all the healthcare institution categories mentioned in this book. The practice of a nurse also depends on the emphasis or specific specialty or service(s) a hospital provides. This means that a nurse working in an ophthalmic hospital or clinic must have been chosen on the basis of having been trained in ophthalmic nursing apart from obtaining the basic nursing qualification. The same applies to centers that limit their services to pediatrics, general surgery, or sub-specialties of the major specialties like orthopedics, dialysis units, and neonatology. Tertiary hospitals have departments based on specialties, so nurses usually work in the areas of their specialization.

Most large hospitals also have out-patients and in-patient departments that naturally work in tandem for smooth service delivery to patients in the various specialties. In other instances, the out-patients department is general and most patients do not go beyond this section except for investigations, collection of drugs, or fee payment.

Planning and monitoring of the work of nurses should be done efficiently and professionally. Most nursing services involve shift work. Peculiarities of shift work should be managed well so that there is continuity in service delivery. One of the results should be a seamless handing-over akin to consistent, successful passing on of the baton during running a relay race. Patients and patients' relatives should not notice a change in the level or quality of nursing care delivery between members of one shift and another. Members of one shift should not be overburdened while those of another shift with the same number of patients work like they have no patients or have significantly fewer patients.

Even small private health institutions require the services of nursing personnel. Some of these hospitals may require their nurses to multi-task by being engaged in areas outside the scope of basic training and practice of nurses. The nurse may thus be required to do some administrative work, be at the front desk, dispense drugs to the few patients they attend to, and carry out some other assignments or responsibilities. These add to the scope of experience of nurses in such organizations, which may not be simply stand-alone small clinics but high-profile clinics operated by (or in) non-medical institutions like banks, oil companies, secondary schools, or university staff/student medical centers. At the stage of interview and selection, the interview panelists usually bring up this peculiarity to the interviewee. The prospective nurse employees may be fresh to the system or have had experience working in similar places. Nurses who are willing or able to function in additional capacities may be the professionals who are preferred for giving an offer of employment. Such institutions would usually carry out orientation and training of the new employees to properly equip them for the additional role(s).

One of the special features of nursing services is that among all health workers, nursing personnel appear to have the greatest or most extensive contact, time-wise, with patients. Be it in the outpatient setting or an in-patient environment, including the various operating rooms (theaters), nurses spend significant time with patients. It goes without much controversy that these near-ubiquitous hospital workers have the potential to create lasting impressions on patients and patients' relationships. Therefore, all nurses must remember that they are ambassadors of the health profession and should use this great opportunity positively and not negatively.

It is important for every hospital management to ensure that selection, remuneration, welfare, retention, professional development, and employee separation and retirement policies affecting nurses are professionally and fairly handled for them to get the best out of nurses.

These are not all the avenues for engaging nursing personnel. Whether nurses are expected to play typical or atypical professional roles, an institution can get the best from its nursing personnel when they do the right things at the right times for the right purposes/goals.

Professional development enables nurses to grow in various aspects of service delivery and to improve their knowledge or acquire further skills to become proficient in executing the demands of their current or future responsibilities. Nursing is not a static field but a continuously evolving one. There are updates for all nurses and various programs in specific areas for nurses who may benefit from them. The programs may not be specific to nursing development; some programs may be on management, while others may be short courses. In the USA, nurses obtain several certifications in addition to their initial license. Nurses are trained to obtain skills in essential life-saving procedures that are embedded in programs like BLS (basic life support), ACLS (advanced cardiac life support), PALS (pediatric advanced life support), and ATLS (advanced trauma life support). Nurses in the United States and in developing countries like Nigeria may branch out into areas of specialization like occupational health nursing, intensive care nursing, medical-surgical, pediatrics, or emergency department. There are other specialties. Training and professional development must work in a coordinated manner to ensure that nursing personnel, their employers, and patients obtain satisfaction.

Challenges

Challenges in getting the best out of nursing personnel lie briefly in these, among other areas: Prospective nursing personnel, client services, young nurses, shift work, retiring and retired nurses, distribution of nursing personnel, and emotional support.

- ***Prospective nursing personnel:*** It is not every time that young people who want to go into the profession of nursing are the right people. This is not peculiar to the nursing profession but it is essential to see to it that admission into schools of nursing is not based only on satisfactory performance in the entrance examinations.
- ***Client services:*** There is a challenge in this area. Every profession must make adequate provision for placing a high premium on services to their clients. In nursing, as in medicine, the clients are usually "unwilling clients." Their relations fall into the same mold. It takes a greater effort to satisfy them than to satisfy the willing clients. Their impression and the news they spread about services they receive may make or mar the efforts and/or reputation of the institution where nurses work.
- ***Young nurses:*** Young, especially new nurses, occasionally lose enthusiasm for the profession, but they are already in it. In Nigeria, they sometimes meet patients who were their classmates in secondary (high) school, and some appear to have climbed the societal ladder faster than them. At other times, some of their nursing colleagues get married to people in other fields of endeavor and their lifestyle is promptly changed and more desirable. Inexperience in life may not allow such young nurses to put these and other circumstances in the right perspective and may affect their productivity negatively.
- ***Shift work:*** Shift work is a challenge, especially for nurses with young families. Where the workload is particularly heavy, or the staffing level is on the low side, it may be difficult to organize the exigencies of work and those of family, social, and spiritual life. The duty shift of greatest concern for many nurses is the night

shift. It is only much later in the work life that some senior nursing personnel with fewer family encumbrances may embrace night shift duties. Young nurses who find night shift duties more acceptable are usually either single or are alone in the town or city of employment while their spouses and children are in a location different from their place of work, especially when they have enough alternative support to attend to their regular family matters – but how many nursing personnel find this to be their situation?

- ***Retiring and retired nurses:*** The retirement of nursing personnel creates a big strain on the nursing services of some health institutions; even the pre-retirement period does. This is because top management may not be able to replace them with middle-class or relatively senior nurses. This challenging situation may arise from batch statutory retirement (in which case nurses who started work at almost the same time and gained employment in one hospital terminate their work lives together or almost at the same time). In Nigeria and other developing countries this situation may be coupled with poor succession planning complicated by a poor economy, defective general planning, and a poorly implemented staff development that does not specifically aim at filling the gaps created by death or retirement. Older nurses may have had and utilized opportunities for training and development at international establishments, but such services have been discontinued in many states in Nigeria. Mentoring of younger nurses by their older and more experienced supervisors may not have been encouraged because there were no obvious benefits to the retiring or retired nurses. Governments, private sector hospital proprietors, and managers of health institutions may have become used to the status quo, ignoring the fact that time would change the good opportunities, thus putting both the institutions and their clients at a great disadvantage.
- ***Distribution of nursing personnel:*** In Nigeria, at the federal level, and in the states, the distribution of nursing personnel and other healthcare personnel is skewed. While the majority of Nigerians dwell in rural areas and semi-urban areas, nursing personnel are heavily stacked in the big towns/cities, state capitals, and where federal government presence is felt, precisely in teaching hospitals. This uneven distribution is a challenge, and many nurses in the private sector and non-teaching hospital settings continue to eye employment opportunities in teaching hospitals. This is mainly because of higher remuneration and a greater sense of "job security." It is well known that the more peripheral hospitals (especially the old ones) sometimes provide accommodation for nursing, medical, and other personnel via designated staff quarters, but there are no additional incentives to work and continue working in such facilities.
- ***Emotional support:*** Many non-nurses (especially people who do not belong to the healthcare sector) may not understand or appreciate the heavy emotional

burden associated with continuously attending to clients who undergo pain and suffering. Like medical personnel, nurses are known to get inundated with work and could endure burn-out quietly, as doing otherwise could be seen as an open admission of weakness. While they attempt to meet the physical and emotional needs of their patients, some nurses also require emotional support. In the Nigerian setting, there is little support arrangement for nurses (the same applies to doctors and other hospital personnel). It is, therefore, not surprising that some nurses may begin to treat patients as objects. In this context, objectification refers to silencing patients or ignoring their concerns in response to the inadequate care or lack of care provided by a burned-out nurse during their shift. Doing so was not their reason for becoming nurses. This is a challenge that may have been hidden or unaddressed for too long. ICD-11 defines burn-out as follows: "Burn-out is a syndrome conceptualized as resulting from chronic workplace stress that has not been successfully managed. It is characterized by three dimensions: feelings of energy depletion or exhaustion; increased mental distance from one's job, or feelings of negativism or cynicism related to one's job; and reduced professional efficacy." [15] American Hospital Association shows that 62% of nurses have experienced burnout, and the American Nurses Foundation documented that young nurses (aged <25 years) are more prone to burnout, with 69% of them reporting it [16, 17]. The American Nursing Foundation recommends to its members and readers preventive measures against burnout to include rest, exercise, and eating well. These would entail sleeping well between shifts, engaging in physical activity, and eating healthy foods [18].

The emphasis on challenges described in this sub-section is on nursing personnel but it is important to note that these challenges reflect the situation for virtually all workers in the healthcare sector. The challenges tend to be worse in places like Nigeria and other developing countries where there may not be any structured arrangement to prevent or mitigate them. The issue of burnout among healthcare professionals and practitioners is currently a global phenomenon. In Nigeria and many developing countries burnout among these employees, particularly in public hospitals, is essentially from overwork due to attending to too many patients. In developed countries, it may be a combination of administrative duties, detailed documentation in anticipation of (or fear of) litigation, or the additional effort involved in staying current and relevant in the various specialties in the healthcare sector.

The office of the Surgeon General of the United States of America states that there will be a shortfall of between 54,100 and 139,000 physicians by 2033 [19]. In developing countries, there is already a greater inequality, with the few physicians becoming fewer from emigration to developed countries like the USA, United Kingdom, France, and Canada. In some parts of the world, doctors are at the risk of leaving medical practice prematurely by virtue of an unrelenting distressing work environment that threatens their physical, emotional, and psychological well-being [19]. Gadzama *et al.*, in a recent study in a private hospital in Abuja, Nigeria, showed that the precarious healthcare delivery status in Nigeria is compounded by burnout. The findings of this cross-sectional study were that 85% of the respondents (who consisted of doctors, nurses, and pharmacists) suffered from burnout [20]. This prevalence among the study population is high. Since many healthcare personnel have emigrated from Nigeria, and others are likely to join in emigrating, it is a matter of utmost importance for the relevant authorities to address the wellbeing of the remaining healthcare workforce. The authors of this article recommended an integration of burnout screening into the health risk assessment of all healthcare professionals in Nigeria.

The Way Forward

As noted earlier, nurses are active participants in rendering efficient team-based services. The training and professional development of nurses enable them to play their role satisfactorily. It is interesting to note that both countries have a stringent institution accreditation process for nursing school programs. In the USA and Nigeria, re-accreditation of nursing programs is conducted every 5 years; however, in the USA, reaccreditation may be conducted earlier depending on the NCLEX pass rates. First-time NCLEX-RN® pass rates are the primary indicator of nursing program quality across the USA. The national first-time pass rate is around 90%, with accreditation and funding risks for programs falling below 85%.

Advanced Practice Roles

In many countries like the USA, United Kingdom, Australia, and Canada nursing has seen an evolution of advanced practice. Nursing specialties at the graduate level include educators, management and administration, clinical nurse leaders (CNL), clinical nurse specialists (CNS), certified registered nurse anesthetists (CRNA), advanced practice registered nurse (APRN), and nurse practitioners (NP). Nurse practitioners are mid-level providers who, in most states, must work in collaboration with physicians to provide primary care, hospitalist, emergency room, and intensive care unit (ICU) cover. A few states allow nurse practitioners to work independent of physician oversight. In Nigeria, according to the NMCN, one of the advanced practice roles recognized at the time of writing is the nurse anesthetist.

Rural Areas/Limited Healthcare Services

In rural areas where there are limited healthcare resources and where nurses are taking on more advanced roles, it is important to consider providing advanced practice nursing programs in universities and other institutions to meet the needs of healthcare services in these numerous rural communities. Currently, the USA provides various national certification examinations that prove nurses' skill set and knowledge level at providing certain services anywhere in the country. Such certifications would be highly beneficial to Nigeria as many nurses already have advanced training, but with no national certifying examination to ensure standardized quality of training nationwide.

CONCLUSION

The profession of nursing is a noble one. Regarding the nursing shortage globally, there are many job opportunities for nurses. Educational programs may be different between the United States and Nigeria (and other developing countries), but incorporating innovative teaching methodologies like simulation, interactive case studies, virtual clinical tools, task trainers, and advanced technological devices would elevate the critical thinking skills of nursing students and prepare them for clinical practice anywhere in Nigeria and the world. Maintaining high standards in schools of nursing and universities that offer degree programs in nursing is a good initial step to creating a solid foundation for nurses and their practice. There should be an increase in the number of training institutions for nursing, but proliferation should be avoided as the latter may lead to poor training if there is no commensurate employment and satisfactory remuneration for such essential personnel. Educational institutions must not deviate from the standard of recruiting and training students who are best suited for nursing in terms of aptitude and character.

Providing excellent educational programs and providing fair and transparent opportunities for advancement within each of the many professions whose professionals team up to provide healthcare services in hospitals, be they large or small, in remote and rural areas or in towns and cities, and incorporating an efficient separation and retirement plan for every healthcare worker would, with other benefits, ensure that a country and its peoples get the best out of the healthcare workforce – whether in Nigeria or in any developing country.

REFERENCES

[1] Salaries of instructional and administrative nursing faculty. In: Nursing Faculty Shortage Fact Sheet 2024. Available from: https://www.aacnnursing.org/news-data/fact-sheets/nursing-faculty-shortage

[2] Fang D, Kesten K. Retirements and succession of nursing faculty in 2016; 2025. [http://dx.doi.org/10.1016/j.outlook.2017.03.003]

[3] Nurse Anesthetists, nurse midwives, and nurse practitioners In: Occupational outlook handbook. Available from: https://www.bls.gov/ooh/healthcare/nurse-anesthetists-nurse-midwives-and-nurse-practitioners.htm#tab-1

[4] Higher compensation in clinical and private-sector settings is luring current and potential nurse educators away from teaching. In: Nursing Faculty Shortage Fact Sheet Available from: https://www.aacnnursing.org/news-data/fact-sheets/nursing-faculty-shortage

[5] Anarado A, Agu G, Nwonu E. Factors hindering clinical training of students in selected nursing educational institutions in Southeastern Nigeria. 2016. [http://dx.doi.org/10.1016/j.nedt.2016.02.022]

[6] Aghedo P, Owoeye I, Adeyemo M, Nwachukwu V, Ogidan O. Challenges in communication with Nursing and Midwifery Council of Nigeria (NMCN). Int J Innov Sci Res Technol 2020; 5(6). Available from: http://www.ijisrt.com

[7] Ojo I, Oyediran O, Afolabi E, Olaogun A, Adejumo P. Making nurses and nursing care visible in Nigeria. A review of standardized nursing care plan from the nurse len. Mediterr Nurs Midwifery 2023; 3(3): 106-16. [http://dx.doi.org/10.4274/MNM.2023.22106]

[8] Ojewole F, Samole A. Evaluation of the nursing process utilization in a teaching hospital, Ogun State, Nigeria. Journal of Nursing and Midwifery Sciences 2017; 4(3): 97-03. [http://dx.doi.org/10.4103/JNMS.JNMS_13_17]

[9] Ojo IO, Adejumo PO, Olaogun AAE, Oyediran OO. Perception of nursing student about integrating standardized nursing language into the nursing curriculum at two nigerian universities. Int J Afr Nurs Sci 2020; 12: 100192. [http://dx.doi.org/10.1016/j.ijans.2020.100192]

[10] Adubi IO, Olaogun AA, Adejumo PO. Effect of standardized nursing language continuing education programme on nurses' documentation of care at university college hospital, ibadan. Nurs Open 2017; 5(1): 37-44. [http://dx.doi.org/10.1002/nop2.108] [PMID: 29344393]

[11] Adereti CS, Olaogun AA. Use of electronic and paper-based standardized nursing care plans to improve nurses' documentation quality in a nigerian teaching hospital. Int J Nurs Knowl 2019; 30(4): 219-27. [http://dx.doi.org/10.1111/2047-3095.12232] [PMID: 30525306]

[12] Zainab S, Salawu R. Determinants of utilisation of nursing process among nurses in University College Hospital, Ibadan, Oyo State, Nigeria. J Health Med Nurs 2020; 70(34).

[13] Ojo IO, Olaogun AA. Challenges to sustainability of standardized nursing care plan in selected tertiary health institutions in Nigeria. Int J Nurs Knowl 2023; 34(3): 193-203. [http://dx.doi.org/10.1111/2047-3095.12394] [PMID: 36205459]

[14] Who enrolls in the CGFNS Certification Program®? Available from: https://www.cgfns.org/services /certification/cgfns-certification-program/

[15] WHO. Burn-out an "occupational phenomenon. International Classification Of Diseases Available from: https://www.who.int/news/item/28-05-2019-burn-out-an-occupational-phenomenon -international-classification-of-diseases

[16] Schmidt A. We need to talk about burnout the same way we talk about benefits 2020. Available from: https://www.aha.org/news/blog/2020-10-20-we-need-talk-about-burnout-same-way-we-talk-about-benefits

[17] Younger Nurses More Likely to Experience Negative Impacts from the COVID-19 Pandemic 2022. Available from: https://www.nursingworld.org/news/news-releases/2022-news-releases/new-survey-data--younger-nurses-more-likely-to-experience-negative-impacts-from-the-covid-19-pandemic/

[18] How to Prevent Nurse Burnout Available from: https://www.nursingworld.org/content-hub/resources/workplace/what-is-nurse-burnout-how-to-prevent-it/

[19] Health Worker Burnout. In: Office of the Surgeon General US Department of Health and Human Services Available from: https://www.hhs.gov/surgeongeneral/priorities/health-worker-burnout/index.html#

[20] Gadzama N, Wudiri Z, Ofoli J, Ede V, Stephen Y. Assessing burnout among healthcare professionals in a private hospital in Abuja, Nigeria: prevalence, patterns, and implications. West Afr J Med 2023; 40: 44-5.

CHAPTER 6

Growth and Transformation of Faith-based Hospitals: Bowen University Teaching Hospital'S Story of Focus and Resilience

OmoOlorun G. Olupona[1,*]

[1] *Bowen University Teaching Hospital, Ogbomos, Oyo, Nigeria*

Abstract: One of the reasons for choosing Bowen University Teaching Hospital as a "case study" in this book is that it is a quintessential example of a hospital that started not with the aim of making profit but to render medical services to a poor and, at the time of its inception, a rural community but somehow survived the intricacies of medical practice in Nigeria and, today, is rendering primary, secondary, and tertiary healthcare services. The services of this hospital attract patients from nearby communities and nearby states in the South-Western geopolitical zone of Nigeria.

This is an interesting story with ups and downs, periods of uncertainty and joy, periods of support and virtually standing alone to believe in itself – and most importantly, periods of taking "a leap of faith" that has taken it to an enviable league of a tertiary hospital that trains medical students, postgraduate (resident) doctors, and undergraduate students in nursing.

The story of Bowen University Teaching Hospital should encourage any hospital irrespective of its ownership to aim for greater heights and to believe that when medical services are rendered from the mindset of running a marathon race and concomitantly satisfying their patients and communities consistently, only the future can tell what a hospital with a humble beginning can become.

Keywords: Bowen university iwo, Nigerian baptist conventionnational health insurance scheme, Ogbomoso baptist hospital, Ogbomoso, Southern baptist convention.

INTRODUCTION

In Nigeria, most faith-based hospitals are called "Mission Hospitals," and the name seems to derive from missionaries who came to Africa (including Nigeria)

* **Corresponding author OmoOlorun G. Olupona:** Bowen University Teaching Hospital, Ogbomos, Oyo, Nigeria; E-mail: oolupona@gmail.com

Impact Clinics Ltd. has since replaced the former company name RST Clinics Ltd.

to propagate their faith, the Christian faith. Interestingly, these hospitals have lasted for more than half a century, and many are still operational although they have been handed over to their Nigerian equivalent or the communities where they are. In some instances, the government in various states unilaterally created laws that enabled them to take over some of these hospitals. The author of this book (not this Chapter) was born in one of these hospitals, and it is still functional. The story of Bowen University Teaching Hospital narrated in this Chapter, is about one such hospital, and one that has stood the test of time and is not only operational but also has been transformed into a tertiary hospital in Nigeria. It is in the southern part of the country. Another hospital (run by another Mission) is in the northern part of Nigeria and has contributed significantly to the health care of Northern Nigeria and, similarly, transmuted into a university teaching hospital.

Concept of the Medical Facility

The Southern Baptist Convention of the United States of America began its mission work in Nigeria when its first missionary, Thomas Jefferson Bowen, arrived in the country in 1850 and started work in Ijaiye, Lagos, and Ogbomoso [1]. The initial focus was the establishment of churches with self-governing congregations. In line with the tripod ministry of Jesus Christ, the mission work was later extended to the teaching and healing ministries. The first hospital to be established by the Southern Baptist Convention in Nigeria was Ogbomoso Baptist Hospital. It was established on 18 March 1907 with the arrival of Dr. George Green and his newly wed bride, Lydia, in Ogbomoso [2]. Dr. Green, who was born in London, was influenced by his godly parents. At the age of 22 years, he left London for Montreal, Canada, and in the following year, he took ill with the flu. He received compassionate care from a physician who was a member of his local Baptist Church and convalesced in the home of another member. These kind acts sowed the desire for him to become a medical doctor. In 1897, he relocated to Woodstock, Ontario, where he met the Sweet family and professors at Woodstock Baptist College, whose parents had served as missionaries in India. These godly people influenced his interest in missions and ministry work. Due to his ever-increasing passion for mission work, he sold off his flourishing book binding business and enrolled in Woodstock Baptist College, an affiliate of McMaster University. His excellent educational background enabled him to complete the course in one year. He was licensed to preach by the First Baptist Church, Woodstock, in 1899 and completed his college education in 1900.

Green relocated to the United States of America having been convinced of a call into the medical ministry; he sought admission and was admitted into the Medical College of Virginia in Richmond in September 1901. He received his degree of

Doctor of Medicine in May 1905. The Foreign Mission Board of the Southern Baptist Convention appointed him as the first medical missionary to Africa, and he was ordained into the ministry on 26 November 1906. He and Lydia were married on 09 January 1907 in Norfolk. The newly wedded couple went directly from the church to the wharf to board the steamer from Norfolk en-route to Lagos *via* Richmond, New York. They finally departed for Lagos on 19 January 1907. They arrived in Lagos on 04 March 1907 and finally in Ogbomoso on 18 March 1907 (Fig. **1**). Dr. Green seized every opportunity he had whenever he went back home on furlough to improve his medical knowledge and skills. He obtained the title of Licentiate of the Royal College of Physicians and Surgeons of Edinburgh and Glasgow after passing the qualifying examinations. The success enabled him to join the British Medical Association in 1920.

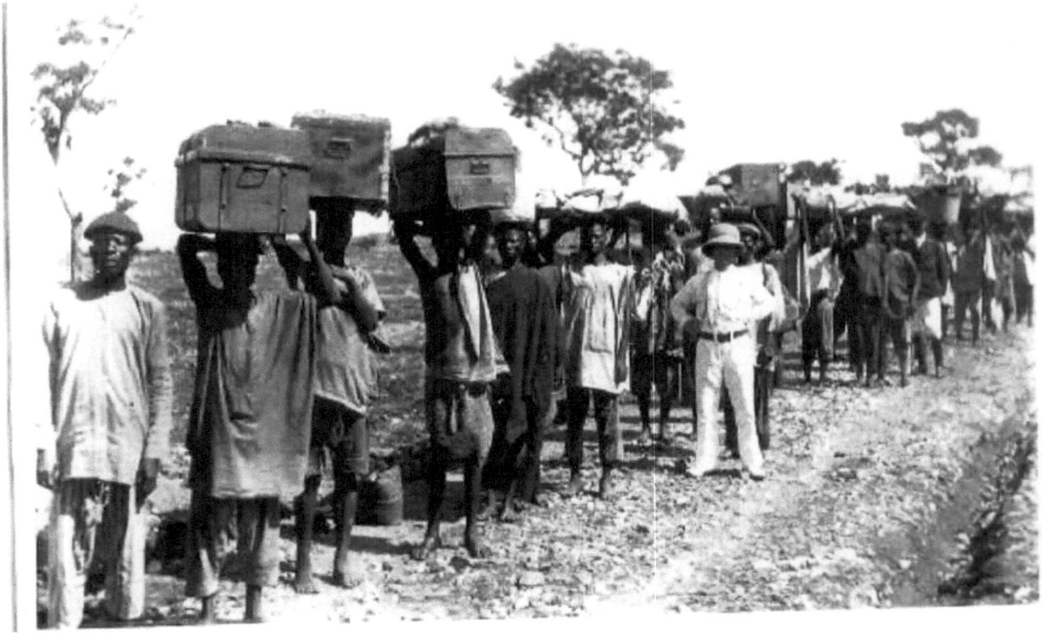

Fig. (1). Dr. George Green and his entourage en route to Ogbomoso (Photo credit – BMC archives).

Over the years, Ogbomoso Baptist Hospital made a name for itself for the quality and compassionate care it rendered to patients from near and far, irrespective of age, gender, religious or political orientation. It became a brand name not only in its immediate surroundings but even in distant places across Nigeria and in neighboring countries, especially where natives of Ogbomoso and its environs had migrated. For 102 years, the hospital remained a secondary health care facility. However, with the establishment of Bowen University Iwo (of the Nigerian Baptist Convention) and the accreditation of the university to run the program for the award of Bachelor's degree in Medicine and Bachelor degree of Surgery, the hospital was upgraded to a teaching hospital known as Bowen University Teaching Hospital (BUTH) on December 01, 2009 [3]. The initial vision of the establishment of the institution as a mission hospital over a century ago did not change. It remained focused on compassionate care and served as a training center for various categories of medical and health workers. Employment opportunities are open to all those who share the vision of the hospital and feel called into this ministry of healing. To the glory of God, members of staff of the hospital have never gone on industrial action, not even for one day since its inception.

Initial Experiences and Growth

The hospital began in the home of Dr. Green and Mrs. Green in one of the mission houses, tagged Mission House 1 (Fig. **2**). This location is the present-day Antioch Baptist Church, opposite to the current location of the hospital [4].

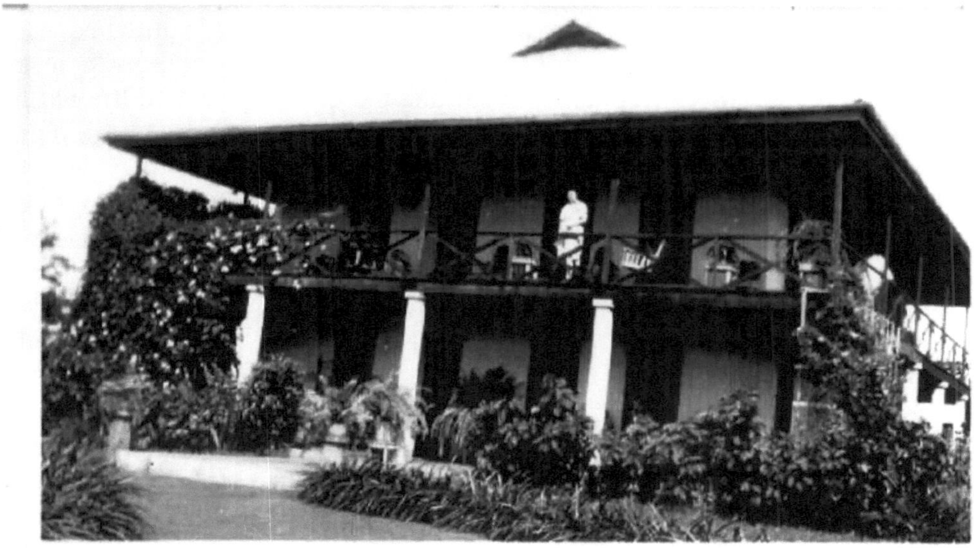

Fig. (2). House serving as residence for the Greens and hospital on the ground floor (Photo credit – BMC archives).

Flamboyant trees in front of the houses provided shade for the patients, and these served as their waiting room. The hospital later moved to the ground floor of House 2 two years later, while the upper floor served as the living quarters for Dr. Green and Mrs. Green. As the work expanded, it further moved to a three-room house, tagged House 3, and thatched roof extensions were built on either side of the house that served as wards for sick men and women. This remained as the hospital for many years until the first set of buildings designed for the hospital was dedicated. The initial work over the first ten years of the ministry was done by the pioneering missionaries. By the second decade, Dr. Basil Lee Lockett, who was in Oyo, relocated to Ogbomoso to join the ministry. In 1923, Miss Ruth Kersey arrived from the United States of America and teamed up with others in the hospital. Mrs. Ruth Mary McCormick, a nurse who was based in and working in Iwo, also joined on a temporary basis from 1928 when Miss Kersey went back home on furlough. Over the next thirty or so years, and by the time Nigeria became an independent nation in 1960, other Baptist hospitals had been established in the four main regions of Nigeria, namely Kotangora in the Northern Region, Joinkrama in the Eastern Region, Eku in the Mid-western Region and another one in Shaki in the Western Region, in addition to the hospital in Ogbomoso.

The Baptist Mission applied for the present site of almost forty acres when the government decided to relocate the rest house and post office across the road from the initial site of the hospital. The first funds for the construction of the permanent buildings were provided in 1917 by the young women of the Women Missionary Union of Virginia, Mrs. Green's home state. Two years later, there was a special campaign by the Southern Baptist Convention, and this provided additional funds. The executive committee of the Baptist Mission in 1921 approved the plans for the proposed buildings. The cornerstone was laid in December of that year. Dr. E. G. Maclean, a dentist who supervised the construction of the buildings for the Baptist College, moved from Iwo to Ogbomoso to supervise the construction of the buildings for the Nigerian Baptist Theological Seminary and the beginning of the construction of the new hospital buildings. In 1922, Rev H. P McCormick came to finish the construction. On 04 July 1923, the Baptist Hospital was dedicated and opened for use.

Those mud buildings were used for 36 years until they were torn down for the space to be utilized for the construction of the initial part of the present facility, which was dedicated on 16 August 1959.

A few of the initial buildings, namely George Green Hall (Fig. **3**), physiotherapy building (Fig. **4**), and a bell tower, are still part of structures in use today on the hospital premises.

Through the years, the hospital has expanded to include other aspects of medical work, such as the training of family physicians, nurses, midwives, interns in pharmacy, medical laboratory science, and dental technology. Others include training of housemen, providing treatment for victims of Hansen's disease and tuberculosis, caring for motherless babies, malnourished children, and providing dental care.

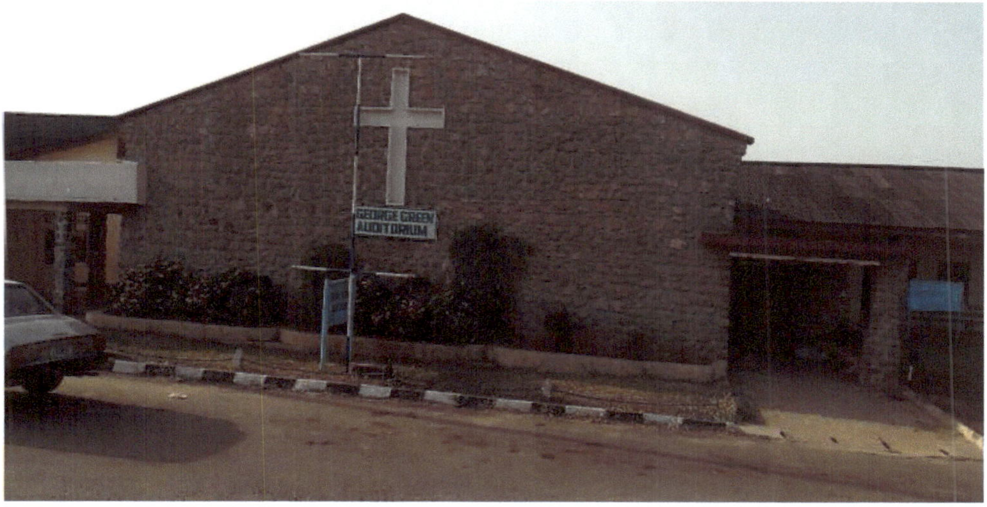

Fig. (3). George Green Auditorium – One of the initial buildings (Photo credit: Dr. OmoOlorun Olupona).

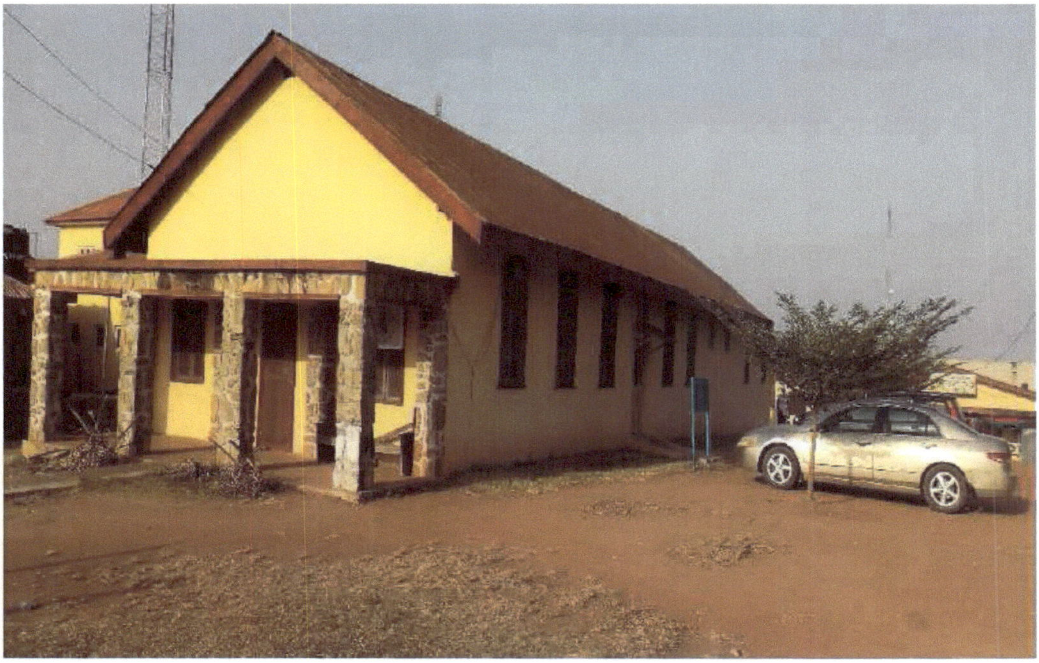

Fig. (4). Another of the initial buildings now being used as a tuberculosis control office and part of the physiotherapy department (Photo credit: Dr. OmoOlorun Olupona).

The Greens' first patient was a little girl, aged about four years, who had suffered severe burns and burn contractures, which subsequently produced significant deformity to one of her legs. Dr. Green converted their dining room into an operation theater and their dining table into the operating table. He brought some personal medical and surgical equipment and drugs, which were deployed in the care of his patients. The surgery was scheduled for the mission meeting time in May 1907. Rev S. G. Pinnock of Oyo mission station acted as the anesthetist. He administered chloroform that was the agent in use at that time. The nurse was Mrs. Lydia Green. The surgery was a tremendous success, and in a few weeks, the girl began to run around in her community. The success of the first surgery on their first patient was a watershed for the budding medical mission. The fame of Green and his new hospital in Ogbomoso soon spread everywhere like bush fire in harmattan [1].

Collaboration with Other Institutions

Collaboration with Baptist Health Service and Kersey Children's Home

Leprosy was a debilitating and disfiguring disease that plagued many people in the early 20th century. In those early years, there were no effective drugs to treat the condition. Ethyl esters of hydnocarpus oil injection were used until the mid-20th century, when one of the sulfa drugs – sulfone- was found to be effective in killing the bacilli responsible for the disease [5]. Around 1930, the native administration provided some funds to set up a leprosy treatment center. Dr. Basil Lee Lockett, a missionary doctor, secured a piece of land about five miles from Ogbomoso town from the *Bale of Ogbomoso* (Soun of Ogbomoso) and established *Ago Ireti* (Camp of Hope). Mrs. Mary Ruth McCormick had earlier established a shelter for patients with leprosy in Iwo. In those early years, the scientific conclusion was that it was useless to attempt to treat any but the early cases. Initially, there was a divergence of opinion between the two pioneers (Dr. Lockett and Mrs. McCormick) of care for patients with leprosy as to whether to admit all cases as proposed by Mrs. McCormick or not, based on her experience treating patients with advanced lesions in Iwo [5]. Admission was limited to only those with the early disease based on what was considered the best practice at that time. However, in 1947, Dr. Goldie was appointed as the superintendent of the health department, and he gave special attention to the work with patients with leprosy [5]. In order to eliminate the strong stigma associated with the disease, the leper colony was renamed as Baptist Health Service (BHS). For many years, Miss Moon, another missionary, was the main pillar for providing excellent nursing care for the patients. The BHS has been closely related to the main hospital since its inception. The excellent care that the patients received over the years resulted in the healthy ones beginning to farm on the large parcel of land that was acquired, despite their deformities. The disease is no longer as devastating as in the last century, as there are effective drugs, and it is far more difficult to contract the disease from those who are adequately treated [4]. Doctors and nurses from BUTH have received additional training with support from the Damien Foundation. Reconstructive surgery is still being offered to those with disability so that they can become more productive.

Another institution that the hospital has had a close link with is Kersey Children's Home (Fig. **5**). In 1926, a man lost his wife after she gave birth to a set of twins. The bereaved father walked many days with the newborn babies to the hospital. Unfortunately, one of the babies died shortly after arrival in the hospital. The missionary nurse working in the hospital at that time was Miss Ruth Kersey. Miss Kersey took care of the baby in her home until she grew to womanhood in a Christian home [4, 5]. She later became a helper in the motherless babies' home. Many more motherless babies were brought to the hospital, and Miss Kersey succeeded in raising funds to provide for the orphans and to build a separate facility from the hospital in another part of Ogbomoso. The first facility was built in 1954 and is still serving till today.

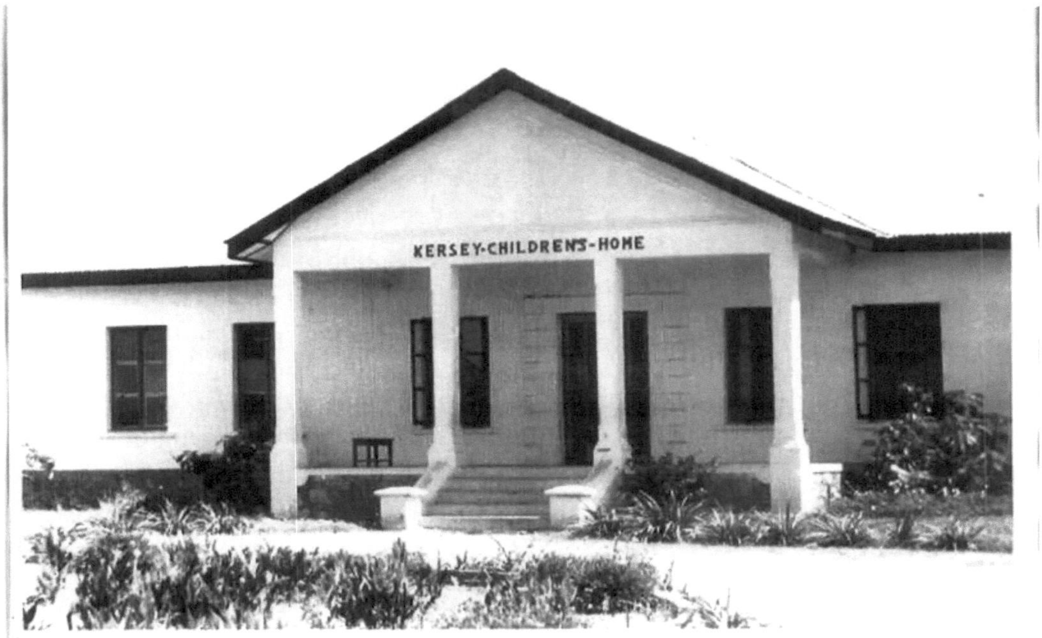

Fig. (5). Kersey Children's Home, 1956 (Photo credit BMC archives).

The facility served for many years as a nutrition rehabilitation center for malnourished children, many of them suffering from marasmus and kwashiorkor (Fig. **6**).

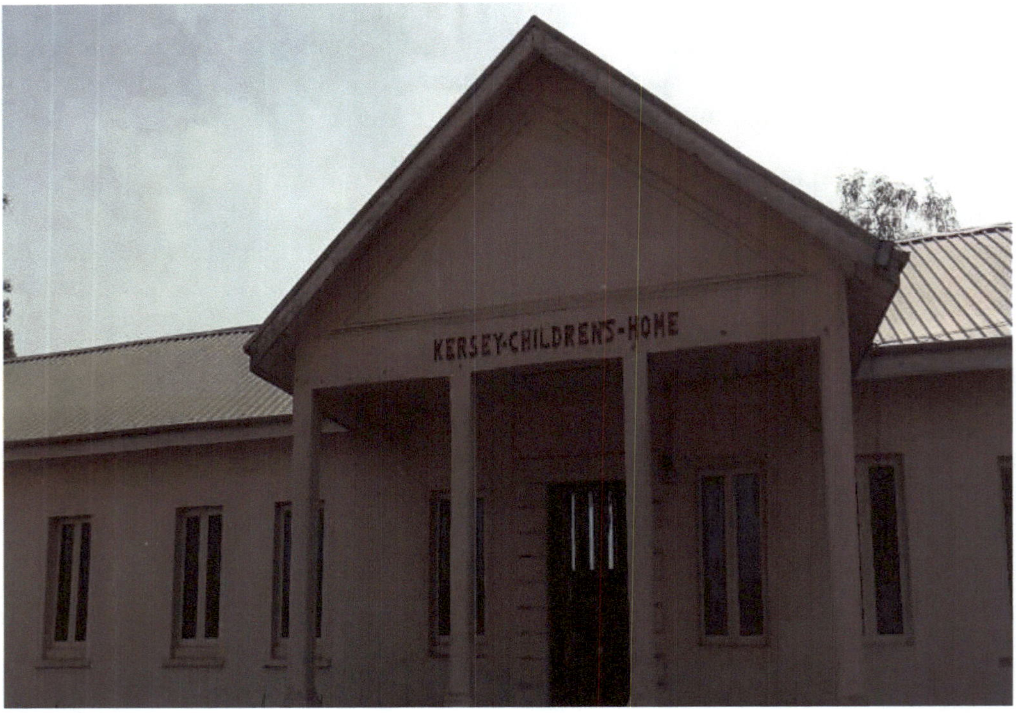

Fig. (6). Kersey Children's Home, 2019 (Photo credit: Dr. OmoOlorun Olupona).

Resident doctors and student nurses from the hospital often rotated through the home to acquire skills on how to manage such cases, as well as providing primary care for children around the home. Soya bean derivatives were the main food used to rehabilitate the children. The mother or a caretaker of the malnourished child lived with the child and learned how to prepare different dishes with soya beans and other important health behaviors that contribute to the wellbeing of the child. Some adult surgical patients who needed nutritional rehabilitation were occasionally sent home. With fewer cases of marasmus and kwashiorkor today, the home cares more for motherless babies. Plans are underway to restructure the facility as part of the pediatrics department of the BUTH [4].

Oversight over other Baptist hospitals in Ayetoro Gbede and Ile Oluji; Establishment of Baptist Hospital, Ejigbo, and Baptist Medical Center, Obanikoro, Lagos

Baptist Medical Center (BMC), Ogbomoso, provided technical support for Baptist hospitals in Ayetoro Gbede in the present-day Kogi State and in Ile Oluji in the present-day Ondo State. Doctors and other health workers were deployed from the BMC, Ogbomoso, to these hospitals, and the hospitals also received support in drugs and other medical supplies procurement. The hospital in Ejigbo was founded by the BMC on behalf of the first five Baptist churches in Ejigbo [3]. More experienced doctors regularly visited to provide additional support and training for the frontline doctors until such a time that the hospitals were able to stand on their own.

In recent years, the BUTH has begun to send consultants and resident staff to provide additional staff on a part-time basis due to the dearth of medical doctors at BMC Ejigbo. The hospital was able to stand on its own for many years. The migration of qualified medical and health personnel has taken its toll on this hospital, hence the intervention once again by the BUTH, albeit for a brief period. The BMC also extended its influence on Lagos by responding to the call of Mr. Hezekiah Alamu, one-time principal of the Baptist Academy in Lagos, for the establishment of Baptist Medical Center, Obanikoro, Lagos. The hospital took off in January 2005. The hospital at Ogbomoso managed BMC, Obanikoro, until August 2015, when it was handed over to the Nigerian Baptist Convention [3]. These steps ensured that the BMC, Ogbomoso, was able to extend its influence and quality care beyond its immediate catchment area.

Acquisition of Equipment and Construction of Additional Buildings through University Funding and Donations by Philanthropists

With the transition of BMC to a teaching hospital after more than one hundred years as a secondary health care facility, Bowen University, Iwo, had to embark on the construction of additional buildings in order to meet accreditation requirements of the various regulatory bodies, principally the National Universities Commission (NUC), the Medical and Dental Council of Nigeria (MDCN), and later the Nursing and Midwifery Council of Nigeria (NMCN), the Medical Rehabilitation Therapists (Registration) Board of Nigeria, Pharmacists Council of Nigeria, and Medical Laboratory Science Council of Nigeria. Since December 2009 when BMC, Ogbomoso, became a tertiary health facility, additional buildings constructed include the administrative block (Figs. **7** and **8**), consultative out-patient department (for the various specialties), accident and emergency department, private, female medical and surgical wards, diagnostic center that houses chemical pathology, hematology, and blood transfusion service laboratories, and radiodiagnosis center [3].

In addition, a pharmacy complex was built; the operating theater and neonatal units were expanded. An extension to the maternity center has been completed following an earlier construction and development of a dialysis center by two families. The same anonymous donor donated the neonatal unit and maternity center extensions. Other new buildings that have been constructed, which have added value to the services of the hospital, include a medical library, physiotherapy unit, and a newly equipped morgue. There has also been an increase in the type and number of hospital equipment that have been acquired. Provision of this equipment has been possible through the support of the university, friends of the hospital staff in and outside Nigeria, and the hospital itself, such as the revenue generated by service provision.

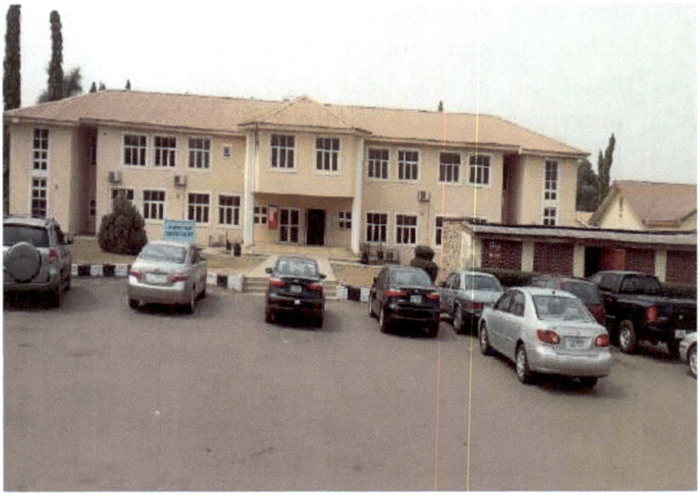

Fig. (7). Administrative building housing the College of Health Sciences and BUTH. Chief Dr. L. A. Gbadamosi was a major donor in the construction of the building, 2020. (Photo credit: Dr. OmoOlorun Olupona).

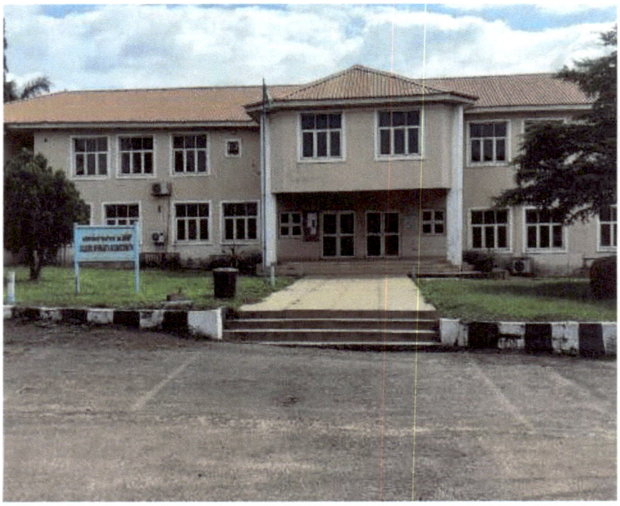

Fig. (8). Administrative building housing the College of Health Sciences and BUTH. Chief Dr. L. A. Gbadamosi was a major donor in the construction of the building, 2024. (Photo credit: Dr. OmoOlorun Olupona).

Governance of the Hospital

The BMC Ogbomoso and later BUTH has been part of the healing ministry of the Nigerian Baptist Convention (NBC) and has been active in the central medical committee and the medical board of the NBC. In the years as BMC, an executive committee ran the affairs of the hospital. This comprised heads of various departments of the hospital and was led by the medical superintendent. Major decisions, for example, appointment, promotion, and discipline of senior staff, were ratified by the medical board of the NBC. There was a local advisory committee comprising community leaders. This committee provided valuable input into how the hospital could overcome challenges and fulfil the mission set before it. When the hospital became a teaching hospital, a hospital management board, which was later changed to a governing board, was inaugurated. The board membership comprised seasoned medical and health professionals, university administrators, financial gurus, representatives of the local Baptist churches, and key officers of the hospital. The board was tenured, and the board under the leadership of its first chair, Deacon Dr. John O Olabisi, was inaugurated by the president of the Nigerian Baptist Convention, Rev. Dr. Samson Olasupo Ayokunle in June 2017. The current chair of the Board is Professor Adekunle David Dunmade, and members are drawn from various parts of the country as described above. The board provides oversight for the management team on behalf of the proprietor.

Friends of the Hospital

The hospital enjoyed the support of many groups. Between January and April 1988, the medical superintendent of BMC at that time, Dr. Peter O Elemile, was sponsored by the Baptist Medical Centers, Alabama, to attend the health services administration course at the University of Birmingham, Alabama. This was followed later by the training of Engineer J B Edowhorhu in biomedical engineering sponsored by BMC, Birmingham, Alabama [6]. Following the disengagement of missionaries from the hospital in 2000, many of them and their children have continued to visit and/or provide technical and material support. One such group is Nigeria Faithful Works (NFW), a not-for-profit charity registered in the United States of America [7]. In 2003, Elaine Neil Orr, an adult "missionary kid" or MK visited Ogbomoso and met with the hospital administrator, Mr. Burster Iyere. On return to the USA, she spoke to other adult MKs who then joined together to consider what they might do. Becky Neil Albritton, Lisa Jester, Jon Low, Harriet Edwards Michael, Alisa Edwards Smith, Lee Brothers Norvell, and Elaine were in the founding group. The fledgling organization began sharing its vision with other MKs and retired missionaries. One of the major projects embarked upon by this group was the drilling of a borehole. With oversight from NFW volunteer engineer Chris Strock and Tunde Adenowo of Sabatek Ltd., the Sabatek crew used a special "rock hammer" drill bit to break through the rock to a deep aquifer of clean and plentiful water in 2005. This borehole has continued to provide clean water for the ever-increasing population on the hospital premises over the years. Another area where this group has provided support to the hospital is equipment such as suction machines and the training of indigenes in biomedical engineering so that they can maintain and repair many of the machines/equipment used in the hospital. For many years, late Rob Dickinson, a native of Zimbabwe and resident of South Africa, was sponsored to visit the hospital to provide on-the-job training for the hospital's biomedical engineering unit staff. Baylor Scott and White Health, also from the USA, has supported the hospital in the procurement of medical equipment and supplies. It is still interested in providing more support.

The support of various friends of the hospital has been of note. Fig. (**9**) shows the Goodnews Kidney Center donated by Chief Dr. David and Mrs. Mildred Ayandiran (building) and Deacon Olatunji K. Belo and family (equipment and water treatment plant). Fig. (**10**) is a photograph of the newly constructed David and Mildred Ayandiran Doctors' House.

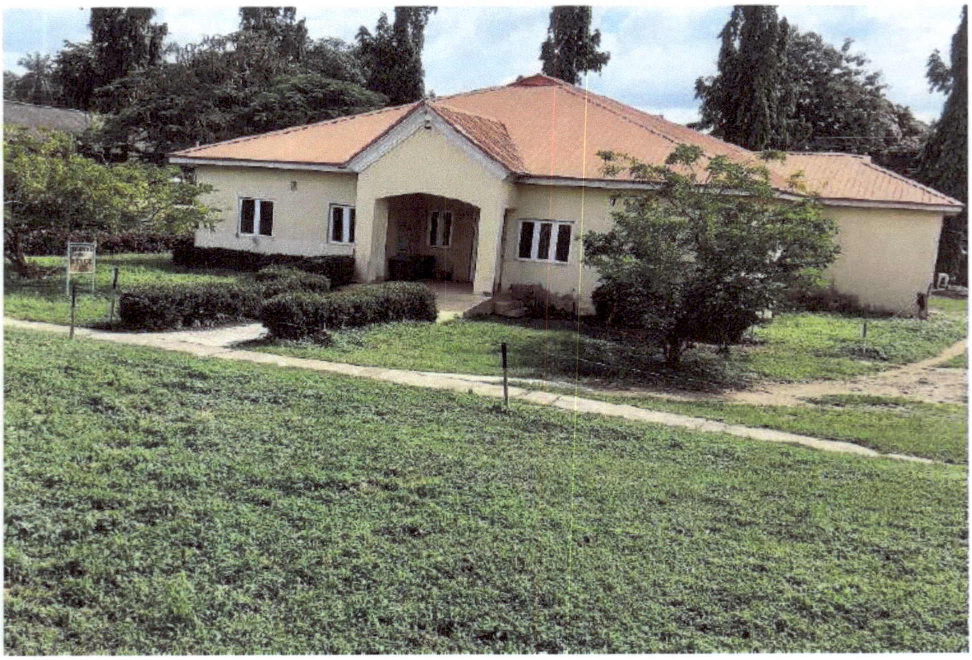

Fig. (9). Goodnews Kidney Center donated by Chief Dr. David and Mrs. Mildred Ayandiran (building) and Deacon Olatunji K. Belo and family (equipment and water treatment plant) (Photo credit: Dr. OmoOlorun Olupona).

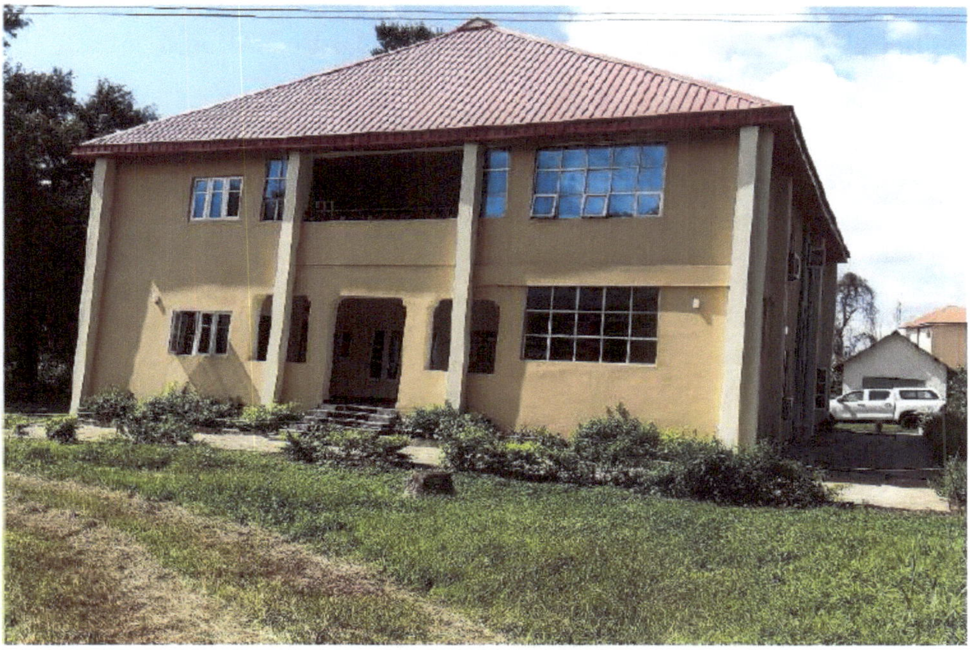

Fig. (10). Newly constructed David and Mildred Ayandiran Doctors' House (Photo credit: Dr. OmoOlorun Olupona).

It is not only foreigners who have been providing support for the hospital as many Nigerian nationals in the diaspora among whom are Dr. Abel Adegoke, a senior/executive partner at Hamilton Medical Center, Birkenhead, and Dr. Olusegun Olujide, an obstetrician and gynecologist based in the United Kingdom (UK) have been doing so. Both of them were trained in the BMC in the 1980s. Dr. Adegoke leads a team of other medical professionals to the hospital, where they not only provide services but also teach residents and medical students, and provide medical equipment and supplies. Dr. Olujide teaches residents and medical students whenever he visits. Dr. Amos Ayanlere, an oral and maxillofacial surgeon who was based in the UK, made two visits in a year during which time he provided care, instructed medical students, and provided medical/dental supplies during his lifetime for many years. Dr. SAB Ogunwade, a professor of oral and maxillofacial surgery, is a Nigerian based in-country who has been providing voluntary service in the care of patients.

Dr. Jire Idowu, who is based in the USA, coordinates the acquisition of medical equipment and supplies on behalf of friends of Baptist hospitals. The hospital has been a beneficiary of such generosity. The support from these friends has enabled the hospital to continue to provide quality care to all who seek health care.

Grants for Community Health Outreach – Ford Foundation, World Vision International (WVI)/United States Agency for International Development (USAID), and Damien Foundation

Over the years, BMC, and later BUTH, have enjoyed some grants from foundations and/or international non-governmental organizations either directly or indirectly. Most of these grants were channeled towards community health care or special groups. In recent years, the Ford Foundation provided support between 1983 and 1998, which enabled the hospital to organize outreach to many villages around Ogbomoso. Activities included immunization of eligible children and women in particular, nutrition education, water and sanitation, health promotion and disease prevention activities, and training of village health workers (VHWs), and traditional birth attendants (TBAs). Different villages had specific days of the month when the mobile team from the hospital visited. During the visits, a team from the hospital comprising the consultant doctor-in-charge of the program, resident doctors in general medical practice (now family medicine), staff nurses/midwives, community health extension workers, and occasionally nursing students, provided growth monitoring, antenatal services, and treatment of minor ailments. Meeting with the village health committee was part of the activities embarked upon. On some occasions, the team brought back to the hospital ill patients who needed hospital care. The VHWs after the initial training returned for monthly refresher courses during which areas of doubt, or challenges they faced in the course of their work in the month, were reviewed with a view to finding solutions to them. It was also an opportunity to replenish their drug supplies, simple over-the-counter drugs to treat malaria, oral rehydration salt to prevent dehydration during diarrheal episodes, analgesics, and other remedies. Sometimes the VHWs accompanied the patients they referred to the hospital based on their standing orders; at other times, they simply gave them the referral slip. Each case was reviewed with them, and if there was a particular thing they needed to do with the patients at their homes, these were explained to them. These visits were avenues to train residents and nursing students in practical primary care at the community level.

Between 1989 and 1997 and with the funding from USAID, WVI partnered with the hospital to expand its reach to more communities, initially in Ogo Oluwa local government area (LGA) during the first funding cycle and later to Oriire LGA during the second funding cycle. Due to the reporting requirements and targets, the Ogbomoso South Child Survival Project (OSCSP) – as it was christened – was not as fully integrated into the hospital program as the community outreach funded by the Ford Foundation [1]. The activities were similar, and with extra funding from the United States ambassador in Nigeria, the project was able to set up income-generating activities (IGAs) for the VHWs, which provided funding to compensate the volunteers for the services they were rendering to their communities. The manager for the OSCSP from inception till 1996 was Dr. OmoOlorun Olupona. It is gratifying to note that in 2024, the VHWs continued to hold their monthly meetings on the last Thursday of the month, and they have continued to sustain one of the IGAs established during the life of OSCSP to provide incentives, no matter how little to the VHWs. Unfortunately, the LGAs have not taken full advantage of these volunteers to promote health and prevent diseases at the community level. Many of these volunteers are getting old, and some of them have passed away. In the first quarter of 2024, they decided to sell off the remaining IGAs – a piece of land and four stores – and divided the proceeds among those who are still alive.

The Damien Foundation, Nigeria, is funded by the Damien Foundation, Belgium, and has been supporting the hospital in the care of patients with leprosy since 1993. The support included training of a doctor and a nurse in restorative surgery and physiotherapy, respectively, in India, improvement in the accommodation of patients with leprosy by the renovation of houses, an old hall, a kitchen, and the construction of water closet toilets with bathroom and a new kitchen. Further support included 50 plastic chairs in the hall equipped with a television set and back-up generator, vocational training for the patients and their dependents, and payment of hospital bills, among others. This support is ongoing as of 2024.

Collaboration with Government Agencies (State and Local) National Agency for the Control of AIDS (NACA) and other Non-Governmental Organizations, Christian Health Association of Nigeria (CHAN), FHI-360, the AIDS Prevention Initiative Nigeria (APIN)

The hospital has been collaborating with agencies of the state and local governments in the provision of care for the general public, especially in the areas of preventive and promotive healthcare. Vaccines for immunizations are received from the local government, and drugs for the treatment of patients infected with HIV and AIDS, and tuberculosis are obtained from the state government. Hospital staff often join their government counterparts during special health campaigns. Students of government institutions who need exposure to the hospital environment during their training (clinical rotation, students' industrial work experience scheme, industrial training) often rotate through the hospital. The students of the hospital's School of Nursing also use some government health facilities for their clinical rotation. The hospital received technical support from FHI-360 and APIN in the care of persons living with HIV and AIDS. The Harvard School of Public Health (HSPH), in partnership with Nigerian governmental and non-governmental agencies and universities in Nigeria, initiated APIN, supported by the Bill and Melinda Gates Foundation in late 2000. The hospital received support for the prevention and treatment of people living with HIV. Other areas of support are reproductive health and tuberculosis control from the Family Health Society (FHS) and the Institute of Human Virology, Nigeria (IHVN), respectively. Support from FHS lasted for a decade and included supplies and training of staff. The support from IHVN is still ongoing, and the installation of solar energy to provide an uninterrupted power supply to the GeneXpert machine and other equipment ensures quality care. The hospital has been an active member of the Christian Health Association of Nigeria (CHAN) and has benefited from the purchase of quality but low-cost generic drugs. The gains have always been passed on to the patients. The relationship has further helped the hospital to fulfil its mission.

Establishment of Schools of Nursing and Midwifery

During the early years of Miss Kersey's work in Baptist Hospital, Ogbomoso, several men were assisting her in nursing care of the patients on a full-time basis, while four girls who were attending elementary school assisted her on a part-time basis of three hours a day. The need to begin the training of nurses became apparent [4, 5]. The responsibility for establishing the school to train nurses for the expanding work fell on Ruth Kersey, Lydia Green, and Mary McCormick. Dr. Locket and Mrs. McCormick began formal classes for men and the first female nurses. The hospital work was organized by Mrs. McCormick, and routines for procedures and treatments were set up. These were compiled into a book form and cards to guide the nurses in carrying out the procedures [5]. Thus, the first School of Nursing of Baptist Hospital, Ogbomoso, was established in 1927. As the Baptist Mission work in Nigeria continued to expand and there were not enough personnel, a plan to relocate the school to Eku was mooted in the mid-1950s. It was not until the end of 1959 when the new school structure was ready that the school could be moved. However, twenty-two years later, in 1981, Ogbomoso Baptist leaders worked hard to re-establish the School of Nursing on the hospital premises [4]. The school has continued to produce highly trained nurses not only for the hospital but also for other health institutions nationwide and overseas. Graduates of the school are highly sought after by public and private hospitals. Many are practicing in Europe, Canada, America, and other parts of Africa.

The School of Midwifery was established as a child of necessity to provide an institution that could continue to provide the holistic training that the School of Nursing was noted for. In order to meet the yearnings of the graduates of the latter, the School of Midwifery was established in 1993 on the same hospital premises. However, with the introduction of the Bachelor of Nursing degree in more universities in Nigeria, the enrolment into the school began to wane, and since the school did not receive any subsidy from anywhere, a decision was taken to close it down in 2018, twenty-five years after it was established.

Challenges over the Years

Takeover of the Hospital by the Government for a Period of 10 Years

In 1972, the military government in Nigeria promulgated the Nigerian Enterprises Promotion Decree, also known as the Indigenization Decree of 1972. This was reviewed in 1977. The Foreign Mission Board transferred the ownership of the hospital to the Nigerian Baptist Convention [1]. In 1975, the Western State government began participation in the affairs of the hospital through the absorption of its staff into government service. There was no change in its mode of administration. By 1979, the civilian government of Chief Bola Ige of the Unity Party of Nigeria took over all the mission hospitals in Oyo State and continued with the policy of making the hospital workers government employees. However, as a result of persistent pressures from the proprietors, the hospitals were returned to their proprietors by the end of 1985, thereby ending a decade of the government's interference in the smooth running of the hospitals prior to the involvement of the government. During the period that the government was involved, considerations in the appointment/deployment of staff were not based strictly on needs; rather, many were political. Inadequate resources meant infrastructure suffered decay, and equipment was not repaired on time or replaced even when they were broken down beyond repairs [3, 4].

Misinterpretations of Initial Efforts to Increase Revenue Generation by the Establishment of a Venture

With the imminent departure of the missionaries and disengagement of the support hitherto provided by them, coupled with the desire to keep the cost of healthcare within the reach of patients who were primarily peasant farmers and petty traders, the hospital decided to establish a venture that was not focused primarily on income from patient care. The lines of business included subletting a small portion of the hospital land to a commercial bank for the establishment of its branch along the main road that links the southern part of the country with the northern part, the establishment of BMC-GORAH Nigeria Limited, and Randa Community Bank. The good intentions of the hospital management were misconstrued by a group of Baptist leaders in Ogbomosho. There were allegations and counter allegations. Issues degenerated to the extent that the warring parties dragged themselves to the law courts, a practice that is unacceptable by the Baptist denomination. Before long, opposing groups arose with prominent Baptist leaders pitching their tents on either side of the divide. The crisis threatened the very existence of the Nigerian Baptist Convention (NBC). As the crisis lingered, many of the hospital's best hands were swept away through irrational redeployments and suspensions by the interim management or personnel resigning out of frustration. Though decisions were taken to resolve the crisis at the business session of the convention in May 1996, a lot of damage had been done while the crisis lasted. The BMC-GORAH Nigeria Limited fell victim to the imbroglio, setting back efforts to generate additional desperately needed revenue for the hospital [1, 6].

Transition into a Teaching Hospital

For over 100 years, BMC, Ogbomoso, operated as a mission secondary health facility. That spirit of being a mission hospital meant that staff members were expected to, and indeed, put in long hours of work at their duty posts. General out-patient clinics were run every day in addition to specialist clinics that were operational at least twice a week. No patient who came for care in the hospital for whatever ailment was turned back, irrespective of the ailment. Whenever patients needed specialist care, they would receive at least initial attention and then would be given an appropriate appointment. The clinic ended only when the last patient was seen, which could be far beyond the regular clinic hours. All doctors, from the most junior to the most senior, lived on the hospital grounds. That meant if any junior doctor had challenges on any particular case that required the intervention of a senior colleague, help was available within a few minutes. Other critical senior employees, such as the pharmacist, chaplain, and head of nursing services, were also residents on the premises. The arrangement ensured that the highest level of care could be provided round-the-clock with necessary interventions available readily.

In December 2009, the secondary health facility was upgraded to a teaching hospital, following the accreditation of the Bachelor of Medicine and Bachelor of Surgery program of the Bowen University, Iwo, by the appropriate government agencies [3, 4]. The proprietor of both the hospital and the university is the NBC, and given the enormous capital needed to run a medical degree program, the logical thing to do was to upgrade the BMC, Ogbomoso, to Bowen University Teaching Hospital. Facilities needed to be upgraded; this was because what was acceptable for treating patients would not meet the teaching hospital accreditation requirements. New buildings had to be erected, additional equipment had to be bought, and diverse medical and surgical specialists and other health professionals had to be hired. As a secondary health facility, the focus was primarily on patient care. Occasionally, medical students from the University College Hospital (UCH), Ibadan, and foreign students used to come for elective postings; the training of students was not a major component of the hospital activities. Research by the doctors was given attention only when there was some spare time for that. These changed when the status changed. Time had to be allocated among the triad of instructing students, caring for patients, and research. Initially, there were conflicts between the old hands in the hospital who were used to a way of working and the new hands who had a different work habit, especially limiting the number of patients that could be seen per clinic session. Patients were also used to being seen quickly, but with the status of a teaching hospital, some delays were inevitable, as teaching of students had to take place, and that required more time with patients. Sometimes, this delay does not go down well with patients.

The hospital does not receive subvention from any government and running costs, including staff salaries and other expenses, which are derived from receipts from fees paid by patients, subsidies from the proprietor and the university, and income generated by the new venture that was established under the new dispensation. The proprietor and the university obviously have limited resources. Barely three years after the transition from a secondary health facility to a teaching hospital, the Oyo State government of Otunba Alao Akala upgraded the General Hospital in Ogbomoso into LAUTECH Teaching Hospital. With an estimated population of about one million people who are peasant farmers and petty traders, and in a town without any industry, the economy is poor, and many patients are unable to pay fees commensurate with the quality of care that they receive. The teaching hospital, being funded by the government, does not contend with generating staff salaries and so is able to charge lower fees compared with BUTH. That further reduces the number of patients that access care at BUTH, and revenue is therefore split between the two teaching hospitals, putting further stress on BUTH's financial system.

Critical Decisions/Actions

Decision of the Baptist Mission to Disengage from the Management of the Hospital

From its inception, the Baptist Mission of the Southern Baptist Convention of the USA undertook the management of the hospital [6]. Prior to 1975, the administration was exclusively in the hands of the Southern Baptist missionaries. When the decade of government takeover of the hospital ended in 1985, its administration passed from the missionaries to the indigenes. Dr. Peter Elemile, who was already a staff member of the hospital, was appointed as its first Indigenous medical superintendent. The Baptist Hospital was renamed Baptist Medical Center to accommodate the transfer from missionary to indigenous administration. During the period of takeover by government and the years that followed, the Baptist missionaries continued to provide service to the patients, drugs, and other medical supplies and equipment in support of the hospital. Volunteers used to come on short mission trips.

In 1990, the Baptist Mission served a 10-year notice of final disengagement from the hospital. The last missionary doctor under the partnership between the Baptist Mission and the NBC left in 2000. That meant major resources that had been available to the hospital for so many years were no longer there. For the years that the missionaries worked in the hospital, the hospital did not bear their costs. They provided free services and also brought equipment and medical supplies. All of these were used to care for patients who did not have to pay; even if a fee was charged, it was symbolic, never the full cost. However, some of the missionaries still return periodically to provide services and also bring medical supplies and drugs.

Establishment of a Venture to Diversify Revenue Generation

The administration of Dr. Peter Elemile recognized the impact that the disengagement of the Southern Baptist Convention, USA, could have on the running of the hospital. This led to the establishment of BMC-GORAH as mentioned earlier. This venture provided additional income to the hospital, thereby enabling the hospital to continue to provide quality healthcare at a reasonable cost to the patients who patronized the hospital, as well as an improvement in the welfare package of the staff [1, 6]. Some benefits, such as a pension that were never enjoyed by the staff, were introduced. There was a time when the staff enjoyed better pay than obtained in the public sector. The additional income also enabled the hospital to provide care at a highly subsidized rate to the pediatric age group, a practice that has been upheld despite the increasing costs in the midst of dwindling income.

As mentioned earlier, this venture was one of the casualties of the crisis that culminated in the termination of Dr. Elemile's administration. The BUTH administration saw the need for such a venture and a new limited liability company, BUTH Health and Allied Services Ltd. was established to handle the non-clinical businesses for the hospital, to increase revenue generation.

Current Status

At the time of writing this chapter, the hospital is in its fifteenth year after attaining the teaching hospital status. During this period, nine sets of medical students of Bowen University, Iwo (BUI) have graduated; the first was in November 2016 after the university secured accreditation from the Medical and Dental Council of Nigeria and the National Universities Commission. Students who were enrolled by BUI for Bachelor's in Nursing Science (BNSc.) and

Bachelor's in Physiotherapy degrees relocated to BUTH, Ogbomoso, in 2017 for their clinical rotations, having completed their pre-clinical course work. The first set of students of both programs graduated in 2020. Despite the economic challenges, the hospital has continued to forge ahead in the provision of excellent care.

The hospital has created a brand name for itself as a result of excellent services over several decades, and, as a result, patients still travel from everywhere (including from the West Africa sub-region) to receive care. The residency for Family Medicine has continued to wax strong. Residency in Obstetrics and Gynecology, General Surgery, and Pediatrics has also begun. In order to minimize the negative impact of insufficient funds, the hospital has gone into partnerships with private service providers, especially in the area of radiodiagnosis. In these partnerships, the private provider brings in the necessary equipment and additional staff while the hospital provides the space, power, and other support systems for the successful implementation of the project. An agreed sharing of the revenue generated is in place. This arrangement ensures that patients receive the best care possible, and there is an increase in the revenue of the hospital, in addition to facilities to further train students on clinical rotation in the hospital. Although the number of patients that are being seen has not grown significantly from the time it was a secondary health facility, the expertise on the ground is more diverse than prior to becoming a teaching hospital. The number of staff, especially medical, nursing, pharmacy, and laboratory personnel, has gone up significantly. Concomitantly, the cost of running the hospital has gone up. While income has increased, the rate of increase lags behind the rate of expenditure.

PLANS FOR THE FUTURE

With the transition from secondary health facility to a teaching hospital, a number of specialties have been added to its areas of service – specialty clinics such as sickle cell, HIV, cardiac, neurology, gastroenterology, orthopedics, soft tissue and bone tumor, and endocrinology. More such specialty clinics are in the pipeline. As a secondary healthcare facility, BMC was among the first training centers in Nigeria to be accredited for the postgraduate training of doctors (residency) in general medical practice (now family medicine). As mentioned earlier, residency in other specialties has started. Many fellows have successfully completed their training and obtained fellowship of the National Postgraduate Medical College of Nigeria and the West African College of Physicians. The plan is to sustain this lofty development and improve thereon and continue to expand its partnership with the private sector for the provision of capital-intensive equipment. To reduce the cost of energy, renewable energy sources will be harnessed to power key areas in the hospital. In the future, the hospital will also extend residency programs to internal medicine.

It is exceedingly difficult for most of the patients to pay the full cost of their care, as only a few are on health insurance, even though the tariffs are very reasonable. Increase in revenue generation therefore, has become imperative. The hospital is accredited by the National Health Insurance Agency (NHIA) and other private fee-for-service health maintenance organizations as a primary and secondary care provider. The hospital has plans to increase the number of enrollees under this scheme. There is a need to continue to expand the facilities as the areas of specialization increase and the university introduces new courses that require clinical attachment. Collaboration with other institutions to maximize resources will be further strengthened, and new opportunities will be explored. Grant acquisition is paramount.

CONCLUSION

BUTH has had a wonderful transition from the secondary healthcare facility status of its "forebear," BMC, Ogbomoso. It has maintained the enviable record of excellent patient care provision. It is also making satisfactory progress in the triad of patient care, training, and research. It plans and hopes to achieve the dream of being one of the best tertiary healthcare institutions in Nigeria and the West African sub-region.

REFERENCES

[1] Ademola Ajayi S. Baptist work in Nigeria 1850–2005: a comprehensive history. Ibadan: BookWright Publ 2010; 19.

[2] Gbadero D A. A eulogy to Dr. George Green M.D. 1872–1962. Presented at the centenary thanksgiving service at ori-oke baptist church on sunday the 18th 2007.

[3] History of baptist medical ministry in Nigeria 1907–2019. Ibadan Nigerian Baptist Convention 2021; 65-5.

[4] Gbadero DA. Ogbomoso: The citadel of baptist medical mission in nigeria. In: D F Oroniran, Esq, Ed Ogbomoso: The Jerusalem of the Baptist in Nigeria; Papers in Honor of Rev Dr Solomon Ademola Ishola, The General Secretary of The Nigerian Baptist Convention. 135-67.

[5] Mary R. McCormick. Memoirs of Nigerian Days 1925-1941. Jackson TN 1981; pp. 90-5.

[6] Ademola Ajayi S. Peter olusola elemile biography of a nigerian baptist missionary physician. Ibadan: BookWright Publishers 2019; pp. 61-74.

[7] Nigeria faithful works. Available from: http://www.nigeriafaithful.org/nfw-history/

CHAPTER 7

The Place of Government Tertiary Hospitals in a Developing Country: The Story of the University of Uyo Teaching Hospital

Emmanuel Kunle Abudu[1,*]

[1] *Department of Pathology, University of Uyo, Uyo, Nigeria*

Abstract: The University of Uyo Teaching Hospital (UUTH), Uyo, is not one of the first-generation teaching hospitals. The story of this hospital is included in this book because it is a story of hope – hope in the sense that with determination, despite humble beginnings, something good, useful, and great can be obtained from something that appears small at the beginning. UUTH was not even conceived as a Teaching Hospital, but the foresight in setting it in a strategic location seems to have made the hospital attractive enough to the Federal Government of Nigeria to convert it into a Teaching Hospital of its university called the University of Uyo. This hospital has adequate grounds that have been fenced to provide security and discourage any form of encroachment. Physically, the hospital has not fully occupied the space available for the small initial hospital. Although it is not as established as the original teaching hospitals, UUTH has achieved a lot and, has weathered many storms and is still standing and getting stronger. It is the only teaching hospital in Akwa Ibom State (an oil-producing State in the South-South geopolitical zone of Nigeria.) The presence of this hospital has helped address the healthcare needs of residents in the 31 local government areas in Akwa Ibom State.

Keywords: Bill waivers, Equipment and consumables, Financial leakages, Firefighting services, Internship, Laundry services, Non-clinical services, Personnel, Renovation, Standard operating procedures.

INTRODUCTION

The University of Uyo Teaching Hospital (UUTH) is among numerous tertiary health institutions in Nigeria established to support manpower development through teaching and research. The target beneficiaries are the immediate community and the proximate ones. The objective of the Federal Government of Nigeria was, and remains, healthcare service delivery in a compassionate and

* **Corresponding author Emmanuel Kunle Abudu:** Department of Pathology, University of Uyo, Uyo, Nigeria; E-mail: ekabudu@yahoo.com

Impact Clinics Ltd. has since replaced the former company name RST Clinics Ltd.

dignifying manner; this objective reflects the mission of all teaching hospitals in Nigeria, and the specific mission that specific hospitals spell out reflects this core mission. In addition, each teaching hospital is set up as a modern health institution that should achieve high-quality healthcare delivery. The intention of the government is to equip each teaching hospital with excellent and modern diagnostic facilities aimed at providing qualitative training, research, and disease prevention.

The Akwa Ibom state government conceived the hospital in 1994, and it was originally called Sani Abacha Specialist Hospital. Clinical services started on January 22, 1996. The Federal Government took it over in 1997 and renamed it Federal Medical Center, Uyo. Following the establishment of a College of Health Sciences at the Federal University of Uyo, a Memorandum of Understanding (MoU) was signed in March 2001 between the Federal Ministry of Health, University of Uyo, and the hospital, making it the University of Uyo Teaching Hospital. This was done in order to enable the students to undergo clinical training.

It is of note that the instrument that accorded the hospital the status of a full-fledged teaching hospital was finally signed on 28 January 2008 by the then President and Commander-in-Chief of the Armed Forces of the Federal Republic of Nigeria, Alhaji Umaru Musa Yar'Adua.

Within a short period after assuming office as the first home-grown Chief Medical Director of the University of Uyo Teaching Hospital, the directorate of clinical services has achieved several achievements that have positively changed the impression of the populace on the quality of healthcare services available in the hospital. These are milestone achievements, though there are also worrisome challenges.

Achievements

The achievements include:

Renovation

The management has undertaken renovation of some buildings for effective healthcare delivery. One of the most significant is the front building, which now has a new look (Fig. **1**).

Other achievements include a new doctors' lounge in the department of accident and emergency, general out-patient department toilets for patients and staff, an intensive care unit, a main theater, a public health block, an old amenity block, medical wards, an old surgical block now occupied by the departments of Ear, Nose, and Throat (ENT), and ophthalmology, maxillofacial surgery, and burns and plastics units. The next two photographs (Figs. **2** and **3**) show how the front building looked prior to renovation.

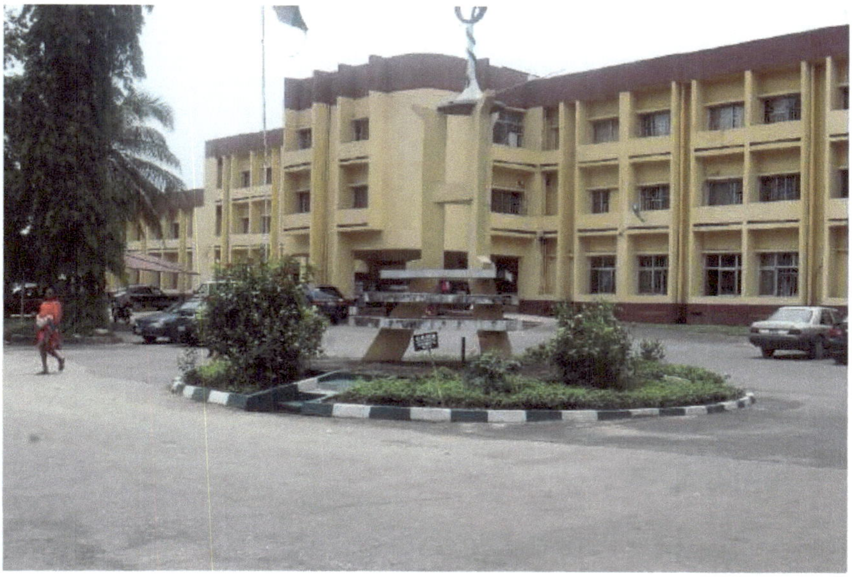

Fig. (1). The front building of the University of Uyo Teaching Hospital, Uyo.

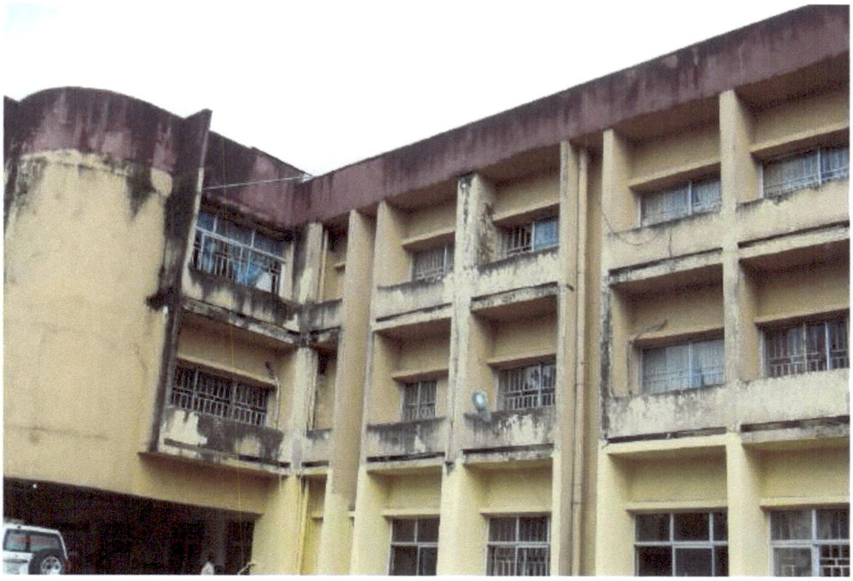

Fig. (2). The front of the teaching hospital (right wing) pre-renovation.

The ground floor of the new school building has been completed to give students of the School of Health Information Management and the School of Community Health Officers a conducive learning environment.

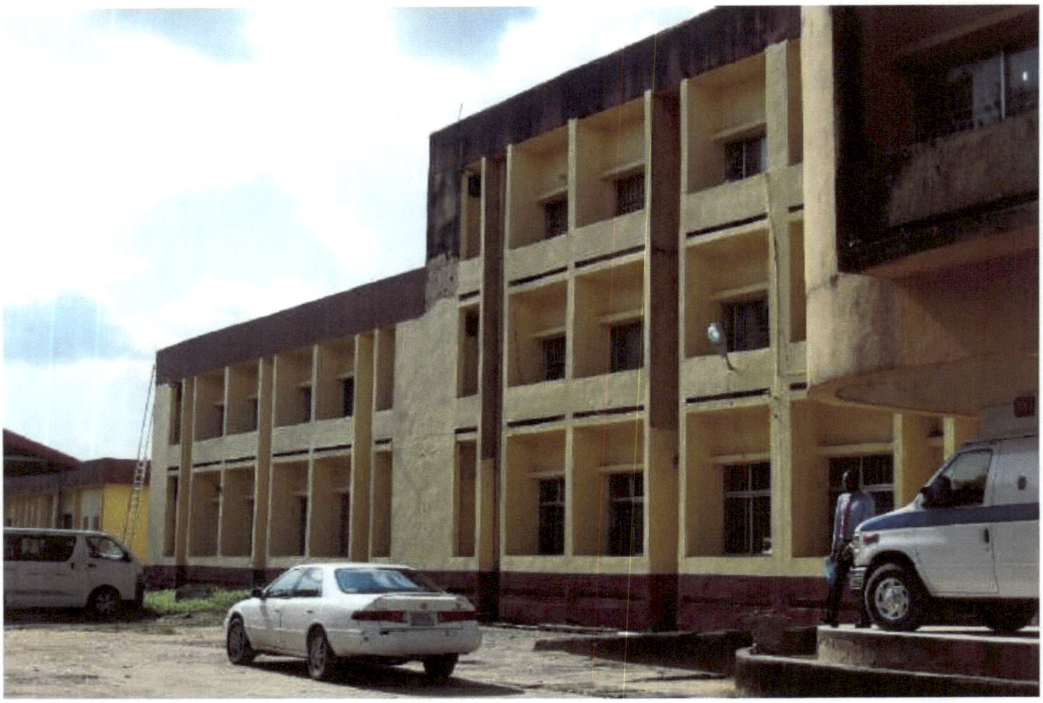

Fig. (3). The front of the teaching hospital (left wing) pre-renovation.

Equipment and Consumables

In addition, the management has provided more working tools for clinical personnel to allow them to perform their duties in the wards and clinics effectively. These tools include dialysis machines. Due to the dire need to give adequate attention to the increasing number of patients who needed dialysis, the management decided to quickly erect a bungalow to serve as a dialysis unit/center. The center has since been renovated and upgraded to serve more patients.

Figs (**4** and **5**) show the building and its interior.

Additional essential tools that have been procured include defibrillators, Electrocardiogram (ECG) machines, autoclave machines, drip stands, pulse oximeters, suction machines, nebulizers, glucometers, sphygmomanometers, and stethoscopes. There has been a refurbishment of Computed Tomography (CT) scan machines, ventilators, and anesthetic machines. More couches have been provided for the accident and emergency unit to accommodate increasing numbers of patients. The new theater wards have also been equipped with seventy beds together with bedside lockers, drip stands, and cupboards. The management of the hospital has also revitalized the oxygen plant, thus ensuring an uninterrupted supply of oxygen to patients in the wards, theaters, and intensive care units.

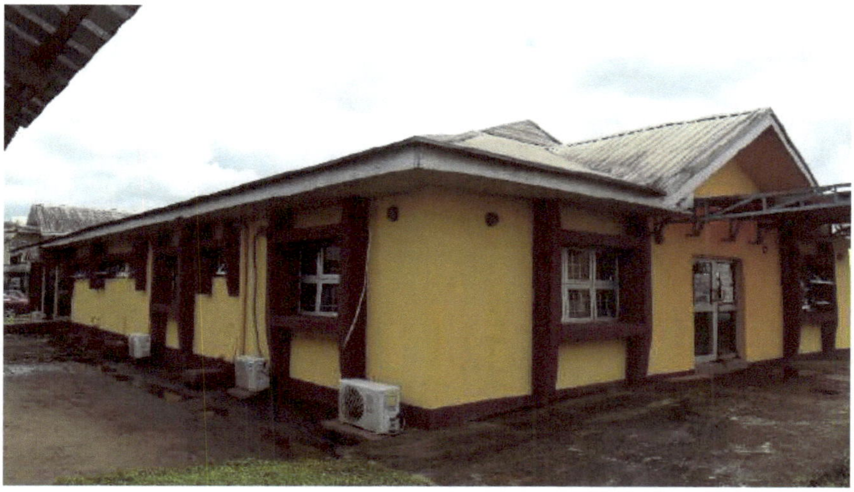

Fig. (4). Dialysis Center at the University of Uyo Teaching Hospital.

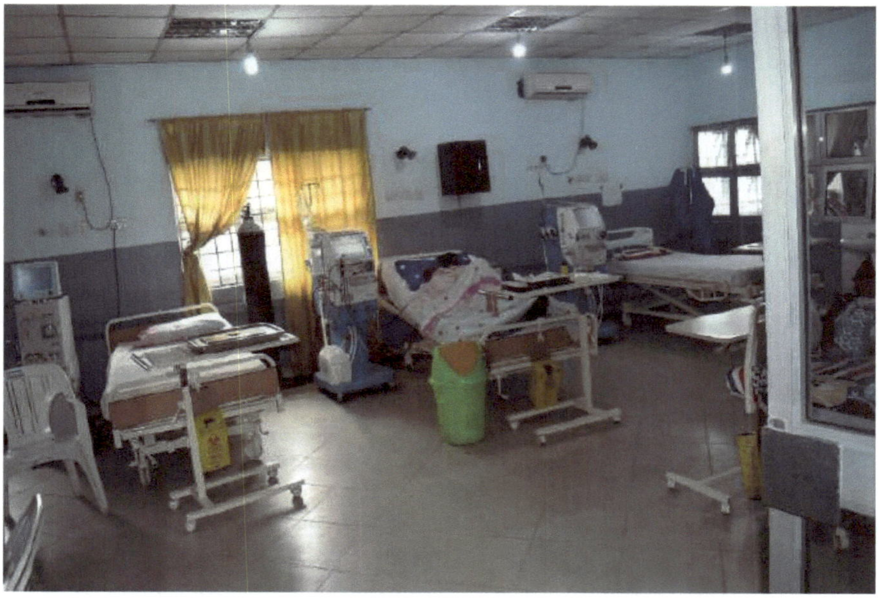

Fig. (5). A ward in the UUTH dialysis center.

The teaching hospital management has ensured a constant supply of medical and surgical consumables to all the clinics, wards, the accident and emergency units, and children's emergency units. This has ensured uninterrupted healthcare services to patients. Additionally, new bed sheets have been provided for the wards. The re-introduction of meals for all on-call professionals has further enhanced services, enabling personnel to better attend to patients with emergency cases.

Academic Activities

Academic activities at various levels have been sustained to ensure that clinical staff are abreast with current knowledge in various fields like medicine, surgery, nursing science, pharmacy, and physiotherapy. These are carried out through monthly hospital grand rounds, quarterly hospital Continuing Medical Education (CME) seminars, weekly departmental seminars, and clinicopathological conferences.

The management has ensured the successful accreditation of the School of Health Information Management by the appropriate council. Daily monitoring of staff, facilities, and clinical activities in the hospital has been undertaken by the Clinical Services Directorate, Clinical Services Quality Assurance Committee, and Service Compact (SERVICOM) unit.

In the Clinical Services Directorate, hospital committees have been reconstituted to help in actualizing the mission statement of the Chief Medical Director of attaining productivity and efficiency within six months of assuming office.

Internship

A successful and continuous collaboration with the Akwa Ibom State government for the placement of medical doctors for an internship (first professional year) program is in place. The University of Uyo Teaching Hospital is ranked second on the Medical and Dental Council of Nigeria's list of approved teaching hospitals for internship training. The number of interns that this hospital is approved to train yearly is sixty [1]. Additionally, management has recruited clinical staff, including consultants, residents, nurses, pharmacists, health records officers, physiotherapists, and medical laboratory scientists to enhance efficient healthcare service delivery.

Residency

The training unit, with the support of management, has successfully undertaken coordinating the training of doctors during residency, thus, promoting a high pass rate for the hospital's residents in the various stages of the fellowship examinations. The Residency Training Program Accredited Institution Database of the National Postgraduate Medical College of Nigeria (NPMCN) shows that the University of Uyo Teaching Hospital is accredited to train postgraduate doctors in various specialties. For example, it has full and current accreditation to train post-graduate doctors (21 at the Part 1 level and 7 at the Part 2 level) in Public health up to November 2026. For Radiology, accreditation is valid until April 2026, and the approval for training is for 16 junior residents and 4 senior residents [2].

Challenges

Despite the mandate of the teaching hospital to care for patients and clients, there are many challenges limiting the delivery of effective healthcare services in our hospital. These include the following:

Infrastructure

The infrastructure at our hospital is old, dilapidated, and inadequate to meet the current growing demand for healthcare services. Many infrastructural challenges have been identified over the years, including inadequate accommodation for offices, call rooms, and consulting rooms. Other issues include dilapidated furniture, toilets, and bathrooms, and leaking roofs. The lack of intercom and other forms of equipment for prompt communication among departments and units has impaired effective healthcare delivery.

Equipment/Instruments/Consumables

The University of Uyo Teaching Hospital is able to save lives despite limited equipment and instruments. However, the available tools are not commensurate with the inadequate number of available professional experts. In addition, much of the equipment for their expertise is either old and obsolete or sparse compared to the patient load; this leaves patients to bear the burden of possible referral to other hospitals within and outside Uyo, which should be rare for a teaching hospital.

Personnel

There is a notable shortage of health personnel across several levels of expertise. For instance, resident doctors who are in a postgraduate training program that typically spans 7 to 9 years often exit the system upon completion or due to resignation for personal reasons. Nurses are in acute shortage; many of them have retired at relatively younger ages since the period of studentship in the schools of nursing and midwifery is counted for them as years of service to the government.

The number of record officers and health attendants is grossly inadequate, thus hindering effective clinical services. Even plumbers, electricians, and other technicians are few and this paucity of personnel who render support services in the hospital cause further harm to the functionality and efficient services delivery by this tertiary care health facility.

Operations

Even when infrastructure, equipment, instruments, and consumables are available, members of staff need to develop and demonstrate the right concept and attitude towards work. It is sad to note that some staff members are not committed and do not have reasonable passion for their jobs, as evidenced by lateness to work, lack of respect for patients and senior colleagues, and misuse of precious working hours to selfish ventures that bring them personal profit.

Some of the personnel at the teaching hospital fail to prioritize their activities. Patients are the reason for the existence of the hospital; recognizing this fact and that their engagement in UUTH is because of patients and ensuring patients' satisfaction at all levels is essential. In some departments and units, the heads decline to carry out effective oversight functions over their subordinates and fail to institute unbiased disciplinary measures that should caution erring members of staff, irrespective of their cadres and affiliations.

Another problem is the failure of consultant pathologists to vet laboratory results as part of quality control to ensure reliable, precise, and accurate assessment of patients' laboratory investigation requests in the hospital. This is due to a pending litigation. Other factors affecting operations in the hospital include a poor referral system, both inter- and intra-departmentally and inefficient communication among health professionals regarding patient care. In some areas of the hospital, the lack of mutual respect among health professionals is worrisome.

There are also difficulties in convincing families of deceased patients to provide consent for clinical autopsies. An autopsy is globally acknowledged as a way to complete the audit on the cause and circumstances surrounding the death of patients in the hospital despite supposedly right clinical diagnoses and treatment.

Finances

Finance is one cardinal factor hindering effective healthcare delivery in our hospital. It is unfortunate that the University of Uyo Teaching Hospital has not received a take-off grant from the federal government since its inception. Poor release of overhead and capital votes from the Accountant-General's office has greatly limited the scope of clinical activities in the hospital. The hospital management is saddled with the responsibility of bearing the heavy financial burdens of the hospital from concomitantly dwindling internally-generated revenue.

There is rising and competing expenditure due to laxity in the drive for revenue increment and unchecked financial losses. Funding foran electronic accounting system, including deploying functional POS machines at the pay points in this hospital, is still lacking. Another strain on the finances of the hospital is the ad hoc payment of cleaners and security personnel from the internally-generated revenue of the hospital. It is statutorily expected that such payment would be released as part of the overhead cost from the office of the Accountant-General of the Federation.

Other worrisome challenges leading to loss of revenue include patients' abscondment after receiving treatment, abandonment of patients by relatives, especially those with some physical deformities, and incessant requests for a waiver of bills.

Power

Clinical activities in the hospital and power supply are inseparable. Effective clinical activities cannot be sustained where there are old power-generating sets that break down frequently. These sets are often overworked, being run beyond the recommended maximum number of hours per day. Frequent servicing and replacement of old parts become a necessity and are inescapable to avoid a total breakdown of these power generators. The current electricity supply is insufficient to meet the increasing demands of clinical services departments to the extent that some clinical service areas with relatively light patient loads are denied power supply for some hours; this is an unavoidable though painful way of stepping down power consumption temporarily. Fig. (**6**) shows a 500kVA power generating set for the hospital.

Other Supporting Non-Clinical Services

Security – Despite the unrelenting pursuit by management to render clinical services in a safe and conducive work environment, the hospital faces a lot of security challenges from time to time. These are due to inadequate security personnel, failure of patients' families to comply strictly with visiting time-frame in the wards and the accident and emergency units, assault of members of staff by patients' families, and frequent thefts.

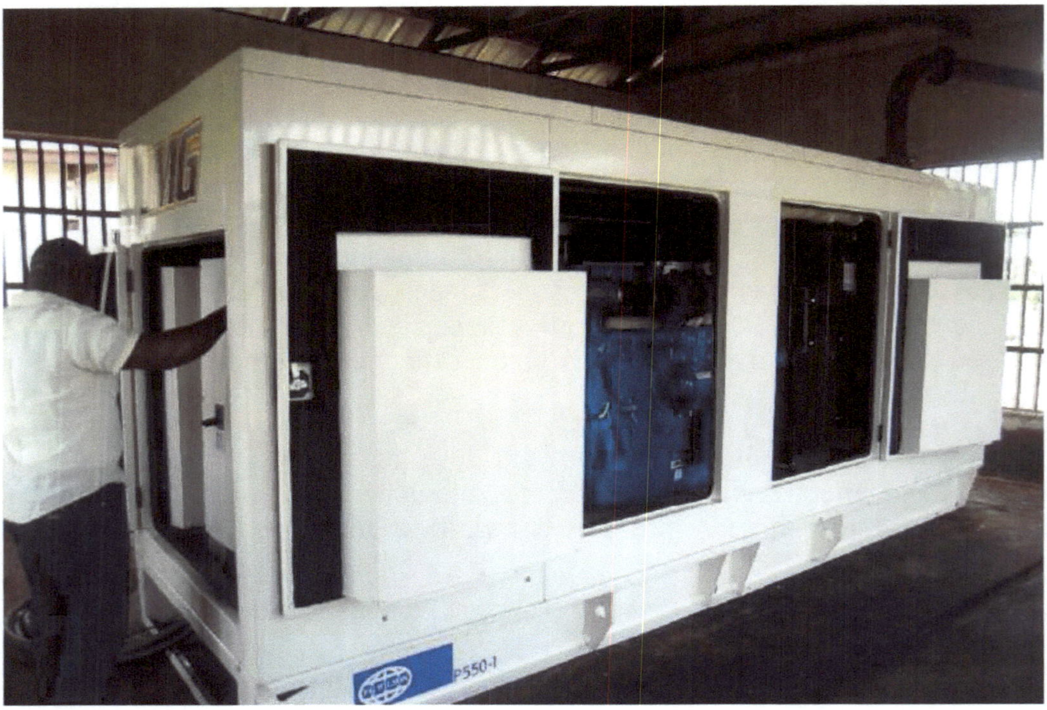

Fig. (6). A 500kVA power generating set for the hospital.

Laundry services – Ineffective laundry services include failure to render services during weekends and public holidays and a lack of washing machines and dryers. These result in laundry staff performing manual washing, which is unsafe, inefficient, and unrealistic.

Fire-fighting services – In addition to the above challenges, failure to have a stand-by fire service station in the hospital does not allow management to meet the increasing demand for emergency preparedness, such as for a major fire outbreak.

Fuel supply – The lack of diesel and petrol mini-stations at this growing major medical facility makes it difficult to meet the demands of running the hospital in situations of fuel scarcity – and this is a recurring issue in not only Akwa Ibom State but also the rest of Nigeria. Currently, the price of diesel is several times higher than it was just four years prior to the time of writing this manuscript

Recommendations to Make Things Work in Our Hospital

Achieving the full functionality of this sole teaching hospital in the whole of Akwa Ibom State and actualizing efficient service delivery is a collective, collaborative, and feasible goal. Both the management and all members of staff (full-fledged employees of the Federal Government of Nigeria and contract personnel) play critical roles in the success of the hospital. Third-party workers like private contract companies, whether major contractors like building contractors or intermediate ones like cleaning service companies, drug and equipment suppliers, security service providers, or minor suppliers of consumables on short notice, all play key roles in ensuring that our hospital meets international standards. With determination and commitment, our members of staff can deliver efficient healthcare services if everybody adopts and practices the right attitude towards work, there is a sustained improvement in funding, and blockage of all sources of financial leakage is ensured.

Attitude to Work

Members of staff must put into practice an acceptable attitude towards work. Cultivation of the right attitude in our hospital can be achieved through engaging members of staff in targeted seminars and workshops. Members of staff who display uncommon selfless effort at work should be rewarded openly to encourage other hospital personnel to emulate this attitude. At the same time, any erring staff must be disciplined accordingly; the objective is to deter other employees who may be engaging in such negative attitudes and practices.

Other attributes that must be displayed by both members of staff and designates of top management are discipline and enforcement of relevant policies. These can be achieved through official circulars to provide information and enhance service delivery.

Principal officers, including those holding offices of accountability, such as heads of various departments or units, must display exemplary leadership; this should include effective oversight functions over their subordinates and punctuality at work. They must insist on responsible officers doing their work.

There is an urgent need to recruit more personnel in areas of gross shortage; such personnel include resident doctors, nurses, records officers, health attendants, revenue clerks, *etc.* This action will reduce work overload among staff.

Management of the hospital should empower and back up heads of clinical departments/units and some top management staff to discipline erring staff irrespective of their cadres, associations, or professional affiliations. Management should also empower consultant pathologists to vet laboratory results in the hospital as part of quality control to achieve reliable and accurate laboratory results.

Lastly, health professionals on shift or call duties should comply with their schedules.

Improved Funding and Blockage of all Financial Leakages

It is paramount to indicate that this hospital cannot run to its full potential without adequate funding from the Federal Government of Nigeria and support from the Akwa Ibom State government, corporate organizations, and individuals who show concern for the health of fellow citizens. Adequate funding would help in providing old and new theaters (operating rooms) with modern equipment for conducting both less specialized and highly specialized surgical operations.

Computerization of Hospital Activities

Computerization of activities in the departments of health information management, finance and stores, laboratory medicine, accident and emergency, children's emergency unit, and the mortuary unit would help make our services timely and patient-friendly and reduce, if not eliminate revenue loss.

Life-saving Arms of the Hospital

It is hoped that when adequate funds are provided, a well-equipped Intensive Care Unit (ICU) will be set up to save more lives. Also, physical expansion and equipping of neonatal units would become a reality.

Salaries of Support Contract Personnel

It is hoped that subvention would be released to the hospital for the payment of salaries of cleaners and security personnel.

Abandonment by Patients' Relatives

Management should strive to put in place strict policies to discourage patients' relatives from abandoning them after treatment has been provided.

Discouragement of Requests for Bill Waivers

It is imperative for the hospital management to ensure a curtailing of incessant requests for waiver of patients' bills.

Infrastructure

Provision of funds from the Federal Government of Nigeria, Akwa Ibom State government, corporate organizations, and individuals can go a long way to remodel or build infrastructure in our hospital, such as accommodation of offices, call rooms, and consulting rooms with good furniture, and more toilets and bathrooms. Achieving this would meet the increasing demand of people for healthcare. The provision of intercoms for prompt communication among departments and units would foster effective healthcare delivery. All abandoned building projects, including the General Outpatient Department (GOPD), laboratory complex, and radiology complex, would be completed, and their completion would create more space for clinical activities. Computerization of all pharmacy stores would ensure proper stock control. The provision of a mini-laboratory is essential for the quality control of drugs. The school block should be completed in order to establish a School of Health Technology with more courses, such as post-basic nursing and technician programs.

Equipment/instruments/consumables

Release of funds from capital vote and special intervention and an increase in internally-generated revenue would assist in the procurement of equipment and instruments to meet the needs of the various professionals, thus extending the scope of clinical activities and improving healthcare delivery.

Personnel

Recruitment of personnel like resident doctors, nurses, medical records officers, health attendants, plumbers, and other technicians would foster effective healthcare delivery.

Power

Procurement of new power-generating sets is necessary for satisfactory healthcare delivery. This should be done through support from the federal government, state government, corporate organizations, and individuals. State and federal governments should sponsor a special and dedicated electricity power line from the national grid to the hospital, thus reducing the cost of procuring diesel for power-generating sets; this could, however, increase the cost per unit of electric power the hospital consumes. The provision of solar power should be strongly considered as the ultimate solution to the current intractable power challenge.

Sundry Matters

Referral and communication – An improved referral system among and within departments and giving timely attention to patients in the hospital must be enhanced to reduce mortality. Furthermore, efficient communication and mutual respect among health professionals in the hospital regarding patient care must be pursued and achieved without delay.

Motivation – Employee motivation can take the form of sponsoring attendance at workshops and seminars, timely promotions to the next rank with the payment of any arrears in case of delays, the release of other allowances such as uniform and inconvenience allowances, and the establishment of a robust and well-structured transport system to transport staff from bus stops near their homes to and from the hospital.

Safety – It is pertinent for management to provide a conducive and safe work environment, which would motivate our employees to increase their productivity. The management of the hospital should deploy Personal Protective Equipment (PPE) appropriate for various employees' duties and train all the workers to use them for their safety and the safety of patients. Establishing a stand-by fire service station and a functional fuel mini-station in the hospital to meet the demands in emergency situations like fire outbreaks and fuel scarcity is necessary to prevent colossal loss of lives and property and damage to the corporate image.

Security – Urgent efforts should be made to recruit more trained security personnel to increase the strength of security personnel and position them around the entire compound. Their distribution should emphasize their presence and vigilance in strategic locations identified as flashpoints in the hospital, like the accident and emergency department, Children's Emergency Ward (CHEW), blood transfusion unit, labor wards, and the mortuary (morgue).

Supporting non-clinical services

Management should ensure that the hospital environment is safe and conducive for employees, patients, and third parties. There should be strict enforcement of visiting time in the wards, accident and emergency unit, and other sensitive areas of the hospital. As already indicated, more security personnel should be recruited for wider security coverage and surveillance; this cannot be overemphasized. Deployment of CCTV cameras in selected and appropriate portions of the hospital would help in improving security coverage.

Laundry Services

Efficient laundry services, including coverage during weekends and public holidays, should be provided. This can be easily achieved through the procurement of high-capacity washing machines, dryers, and necessary consumables, as well as ensuring a regular supply of high-quality water.

Public-private partnership unit – The hospital's public-private partnership unit should source more support from corporate bodies and individuals to boost healthcare delivery in the hospital.

Standard operating procedures – All workers in the hospital should adhere to their professional standard operating procedures for the benefit of patients.

CONCLUSION

In conclusion, our hospital management and workers can work diligently to fulfill their mandate of saving lives through a collective commitment to performing at their best in a safe, motivating, and conducive work environment. This can be achieved with the provision of adequate and regular funding from governments, corporate organizations, and individuals.

REFERENCES

[1] Medical and Dental Council of Nigeria (MDCN). Teaching Hospitals Approved By The Medical And Dental Council Of Nigeria For Internship Training (With Number Of Approved Interns). Available from: https://www.mdcnigeria.org/education/internship-training/

[2] National Postgraduate Medical College of Nigeria (NPMCN). Residency Training Program Accredited Institution Database Available from: https://npmcn.edu.ng/residency-training-program-accredited-institution-database/

CHAPTER 8

Targeted Specialist Medical Services by Private Hospitals: The Mother and Child Hospital Story

Raphael Sunday Olarewaju[1,*]

[1] *Mother and Child Hospital, Lagos, Nigeria*

Abstract: The purpose of including Mother and Child Hospital is to show how a private hospital can provide essential and targeted medical services to patients who reside near and far from it. Mother and Child Hospital is neither a small nor a large hospital but, being a medium-size medical facility, it sits comfortably in-between these two types of hospitals. Like many small and medium-sized hospitals that are set up primarily for profit in addition to rendering medical services, this hospital is situated in the mainland part of Lagos State which is suitable for easy physical access to and financial affordability for its target population – mainly the middle class. The hospital started as an obstetrics and gynecology cum pediatrics outfit and has maintained this target as its clientele.

The story is brief and it demonstrates that any focused medical practice that operates with excellence and patience eventually makes a mark on its patients and patients' relatives. The word of mouth by beneficiaries of medical services in any hospital, especially in private hospitals, is so important that it can make or mar an upcoming or an established hospital. This hospital has been on the right side of history and patronage of its patients. Following the example of this hospital is a recipe for comprehensive success.

Keywords: Financial institutions, Gynecology, Health insurance, Infrastructural needs, Medical investors, Medical practice, Pediatrics, Regulatory agency, Traditional medical practice.

INTRODUCTION

As fact-checked by the editors of Encyclopaedia Britannica, a hospital is "An institution that is built, staffed, and equipped for the diagnosis of disease; for the treatment, both medical and surgical, of the sick and the injured; and for their housing during this process. The modern hospital also often serves as a centre for investigation and for teaching" [1, 2]. It is a place in which the sick and injured

[*] **Corresponding author Raphael Sunday Olarewaju:** Mother and Child Hospital, Lagos, Nigeria; E-mail: ralpholarewaju@yahoo.com

[#] *Impact Clinics Ltd. has since replaced the former company name RST Clinics Ltd.*

are received and treated. A public or private institution founded for reception and cure or the refuge of persons diseased in body or mind or disabled or dependent. A hospital is a place where they are catered for either at their own expense or, more often, by government or charity. It is a place of succor for the sick, the infirm or the unhealthy.

In light of the above, many hospitals in Nigeria today are far from what hospitals should be. Nowadays, most of the medical centers in Nigeria are worse than what General Muhammadu Buhari described as "mere Consulting Clinics" when the Military took over power from the Civilian government in 1983 [3, 4].

The challenge today is how to get our hospitals working again. How do we make our health system become the envy of the world again? How do we attract foreign nationals to our hospitals instead of the current deplorable and unacceptable situation where Nigerians suffer undue hardships and also spend billions of foreign currency on medical tourism annually?

Furthermore, how can entrepreneurial doctors and investors in medicine ensure that they have good medical practice in terms of impact, profitability, and sustainability?

Opening and managing a medical practice can be very exciting and rewarding as owners and operators can make a positive influence on the community they serve while doing what they love. However, entrepreneurial doctors and other medical investors should be mindful of the fact that managing hospitals is also very complex and challenging. Establishing and managing medical concerns are also capital intensive while the returns are usually in trickles but may be enjoyed over a long period. Medical Services are not financial fast-track areas where investors can recoup their investments quickly. This is because medicine and medical practice are mostly seen as human rights and social service issues and everyone or every government involved feels the exorbitant capital outlay.

Medical practitioners by training are usually versed in the science of medicine but may be deficient in the business of medical practice. Establishing and managing a medical practice is a business and the uninitiated should not venture therein without relevant training and experience.

For many doctors who desire to combine medical practice with the business of medicine, the challenge is how to marry their clinical acumen with the management of business, finance, human and material resources to produce a successful and profitable medical practice. How should medical entrepreneurs manage the ever present problems of inadequate infrastructure, medical personnel and finance in developing countries?

It is this arduous task that I attempt to perform using my experience as a specialist medical doctor, a medical educator, and pioneer medical director of a successful private medical concern in Nigeria. The hope is that this modest effort will be useful to those who are bothered by the current deplorable state of our hospitals and want to contribute their quota to right this wrong.

Hospital establishment and management are very expensive and demanding projects that should not be undertaken with levity and unadvisedly. Some of the experiences that have been very helpful in our practice are highlighted in this chapter. It is necessary to reiterate that much of what follows was learned on the job after the commencement of the operation of Mother and Child Hospital (MCH). Because medical students do not learn medical business in schools, many doctors literally jump into medical business with little or no knowledge or experience about business. The lack of knowledge or adequate preparation makes many doctors struggle and labor without success. There is a world of difference between the medical management of diseases and infirmities and the business side of medicine.

The establishment of MCH is a life-long vision that was pursued with all vigor and determination till the commencement of operations in October 1996. The visioner was trained in one of the foremost medical schools in Nigeria. He had a post-graduate qualification in Obstetrics and Gynecology and was a Fellow of the West African College of Surgeons in the Faculty of Obstetrics and Gynecology. He was a medical educator and a consultant to a teaching hospital for years.

The business aspect of medicine was taken care of by working as a staff of a prestigious medical practice in Lagos where he rose to the position of Clinical Director and Consultant Obstetrician and Gynecologist. He attended a management course organized by Centre for Management Development and has a Certificate in Leadership and Management in Health from the University of Washington's distant learning program.

The following suggestions are some important but non-exhaustive factors that should be taken into consideration before any intending medical entrepreneur embarks on the voyage of establishing and managing a medical practice.

The Reason for Starting a Hospital

It is of utmost importance that one sets out clearly why one desires to establish and run a medical facility. Many practitioners would have fared better working in the public or government sector or with an already established practice instead of establishing their own medical practice. Jumping into the fray without counting the cost may bring a lot of regrets later on.

One may ask if it is because you are a medical practitioner and you love to be a medical director? Are you a businessman and just want a more profitable venture? These are not the prerequisites to establish and manage a successful hospital. The above desires can be achieved without the hassles of hospital ownership.

Medicine is mostly perceived as a humanitarian and social service business. Medical practice is a calling. It is the love for humanity and aversion to human suffering that should motivate the "called" to rise to the occasion. You cannot serve God through humanity and serve mammon, the god of money, at the same time. However, a good medical practice will ultimately attract good clientele, which will, in turn, bring about rewarding financial returns, whereas a poor practice will never attract quality patronage. The experience of MCH clearly shows that it pays to start well and stay the course. Commensurate financial rewards are around the corner if one can pay the price and stay the course.

The Target Social Class/Clientele

What kind of medical clients does the hospital aim to attract? You cannot afford to be a jack of all trades and master of none in this time and age, except one who wants to run a primary care medical practice. The clients or social class that the hospital desires to attract will largely determine the location of the facility, the specialty, the equipment needed, the caliber of staff and the financial requirement needed.

It is of utmost importance nowadays that one starts from the area of strength, except the hospital is in a rural area, a primary care center or a general practice.

Mother and Child Hospital started with a bias towards women and children in order to leverage the specialties of the two pioneer senior doctors who were consultant Obstetricians/ Gynecologists and Pediatricians. Mothers and their children are the weak and vulnerable members of the family. Good fathers will do anything to keep their families healthy. The practice has carved a niche for itself as a specialist center for women and children, a place where fathers have peace of mind to cater to the health of the family. The initial focus gave the hospital the opportunity to upgrade the services to specialist areas like Neonatal Intensive Care, Assisted Reproductive Techniques (IVF and ET) and minimally invasive surgeries for women.

Currently, we have expanded the services to other medical specialties and the male gender. This is to make MCH "A one stop family friendly medical center." After all, the fathers are the children of their mothers also; making the name appropriate for all.

It is also necessary to consider the socio-economic status of the clients the hospital wishes to attract. This has a lot to do with the location of your practice, your expected initial financial requirement and quality of the staff. If you pitch your tent to the wealthy only, you may struggle to have enough clients to keep your practice afloat until the facility is fully established. Similarly, in a developing country like Nigeria, the wealthy live in the exclusive and expensive part of the community where financial requirements to purchase land and erect hospitals may be prohibitive. On the other hand, if your practice is mainly for the economically disadvantaged, a lot of your patients may not be able to pay for your services. It is advisable to aim for the middle class at the beginning and gradually upgrade as the practice grows and becomes more acceptable to the people. This was what Mother and Child Hospital did because of the limited available finance and this has largely paid off.

The Available Infrastructure

One needs to assess the infrastructure that is available in the locality before venturing out. It is difficult for a practice to survive and thrive without making use of some basic infrastructure like roads, transportation, water supply, and electricity. You must remember you are not running a government but you need the government to provide some basic amenities before you can run a successful business.

In some rural areas and parts of some cities, running a medical practice is like running a local government because of the dearth of basic infrastructure. This makes the cost of running a successful and profitable business very difficult. Care must be taken so that one does not unwittingly enter unnecessary debt. You must look before you leap.

Sometimes, it may be necessary to consult the local government, the community development associations, or the traditional rulers in the designated area before one begins to put structure in place. These consultations will allow you to know what to expect or how to navigate the problems that may arise in your new locality.

The Available Financial Resource/Funding

It is very important to decide how you will fund your start-up medical practice. If you do not have adequate funds to finance the entire venture yourself, you may have to borrow funds or sell equity.

For a medical practice, it might not be advisable to borrow from banks or other financial institutions in Nigeria nowadays. This is because Nigerian banks usually lend for short tenure but charge high interest rates. Good medical practices involve a long tenure of operation with funds coming in a little at a time. Government facilities are not of much help in our experience. What the Federal government presented as single-digit interest rates to ease the burden of finance in the health sector had been handed over to commercial banks who in turn introduced all sorts of stumbling blocks to block disbursements of the facilities.

One might decide to sell equity but be sure to partner with trustworthy individuals who will not stampede you for quick returns at the expense of good medical practice. Investors and financiers are usually in a hurry to expect returns on investments. Of course, they are right, but financial returns in medicine are not fast track. Doctors and medical investors need to engage legal and financial experts for professional advice in these areas.

Mother and Child Hospital weathered the storm of initial capital and running costs by starting small and growing organically. The practice was started by two shareholders who were friends. The initial capital was provided by an engineer businessman investor, while the visioner medical doctor provided some medical equipment and the expertise. Both of them were willing to sacrifice financial returns for the first few years for the growth of the hospital. The money made in the first few years was mostly used to equip the hospital and attract quality staff.

It is of utmost importance that proper financial accountability and discipline be instituted from the commencement of operations. The bane of most private medical practices is that the manager does not separate his/her personal finance from the finance of the business. Proper financial management was put in place at the beginning of operations in MCH. The visioner, who was the Medical Director/CEO was on salary from the commencement of the hospital. Also, proper account records were kept and an external auditor was available to check the account records regularly.

It was only once that Mother and Child Hospitals ventured into the Nigerian financial or banking sector. A facility of one million Naira was taken to purchase a 40 kVA generator for the hospital. The loan facility was paid-off a few months later when the interest rate was unilaterally reviewed upwards by the bank. The bank claimed that the cost of funds had gone up. Twice, a-single digit interest rate facility awarded to MCH by the Central Bank of Nigeria and recently by the Bank of Industries was not accessed due to very unreasonable demands by the commercial banks through which the loans were to be disbursed. MCH is not indebted to any financial institution anywhere. On many occasions, MCH had been fortunate to receive assistance from the Board in areas of business and financial management and support.

However, the policy of not borrowing to finance the business may not work in some cases. Every business concern needs some financial support at different times and for different purposes. What is of utmost importance is to be clear-headed at all times, avoid high interest rates and short term facilities and utilize the money raised judiciously to avoid undue pressure on the practice. Professional advice from financial and management experts may not be out of place before your business is saddled with avoidable debts.

There are international financial institutions that may assist in the funding of medical start-ups and upgrade of medical facilities. The problem is that these facilities may not be accessible to the uninitiated or the ones not well connected. Thanks be to God; many big and modern private hospitals are being established in different areas of our nation nowadays. These are money-guzzling medical facilities and must require international financial backing or diaspora funding. We hope that these facilities will bring the necessary financial returns to encourage more funding for medical infrastructures in Nigeria.

Ownership and Management Structure

It is commonly said that in life, if you want to go fast, you go alone but if you want to go far, you must go with other people. This is very true as a tree cannot make a forest.

Many practitioners desire to own their own medical practice. This ambition is good and comes with many advantages. However, MCH has greatly benefitted from the advantages of joint ownership and management.

The management board was made up of the joint owners serving as the Chairman and the MD/CEO respectively. The board was later expanded to accommodate three other board members who all have at least 5% shares of the hospital business. The board is the highest decision-making body for the hospitals. Mother and Child Hospital has benefited immensely from the wealth of experience of the board.

The second level of decision making is hospital management, made up of heads of departments/ units and doctors of consultant level under the leadership of the MD/CEO. The groups have made invaluable contributions to the development and growth of Mother and Child Hospitals.

Some years ago, I had the opportunity to attend a business seminar outside Nigeria where ownership and boards of highly successful global companies were discussed. It was concluded that joint ownership with few like–minded people as board members performed far better than the one-man or family-owned businesses. I was glad that MCH adopted the policy from its inception.

Human and Material Resources

The most important resource in any organization is the human resource – the human capital. You will need to put together a good team. To this end, you need to attract and retain relevant professionals who will help manage and run the practice smoothly, efficiently and profitably. You must always remember that you now wear the toga of a medical practitioner and also a manager of people and resources. You also have the board and investors in your business to report to. The realization that you are responsible to some other authority should keep you in line and remind you to put some checks and balances in place every day. This will enable you to manage human and material resources efficiently and profitably. In your daily activities, be sure to consider the following:

- You must continue to learn, update and keep abreast of new discoveries or developments in your profession, business and management. You cannot afford to become obsolete and expose yourself to unnecessary embarrassment or even litigation.
- Be sure to communicate the vision and mission of your practice or business to your staff so that they can run with the vision also, Hab 2: 2 (6). You cannot afford to be a lone ranger or an island of visioners in the midst of the blind.
- Training and re-training must be your top priority to help your staff to adjust to the new environment. MCH commenced a fortnightly Clinical meetings in the hospital few months after the commencement of operations. Staff from different departments were required to give lectures on various topics, share difficult cases and challenges and teach the latest developments about the topics. The meetings were moderated by the heads of units and consultants. Experts from outside the hospitals are usually invited as resource persons to these meetings. Train and retrain until the staff imbibe the vision of your business.
- Infrastructure and equipment: You need to obtain or have access to the right type of equipment, including hospital, laboratory and other specialized equipment. There must be a reliable water supply, reliable power sources, and a reliable supply of pharmaceuticals. There must be a reliable and efficient mechanism to distribute resources and expertise to those in need - especially in the context of infrastructural deficiency in Nigeria today.
- Partnerships and advances in medicine: You will need to engage with colleagues and other medical professionals to create productive partnerships and stay in contact with relevant medical bodies that are involved in training, research, and advocacy.

These resources will help you and your practice to grow, stay relevant, and be abreast with new developments.

Regulating Authority/Government Policies

As with other businesses, government policies can greatly impact your medical practice. In Nigeria, government policy is generally fickle and sometimes changes from one government to the next, and this can sometimes lead to unintended consequences. Take the issue of bank loan, for instance; if the government increases the base rate, commercial banks will also increase the interest rate for any loan taken and your practice might not be able to cope. Also, governments control the regulatory bodies and institutions for medical practice and training. Policies that affect the general medical profession of the country will inevitably affect your private practice, too. These may include policies about pharmaceuticals, health insurance, orthodox, alternative, and traditional medical practices. You should be mindful of all such policies to enable you to practice within the law.

You must spare no efforts to register your practice and maintain cordial relationships with the regulating agencies of governments. You must be abreast of the requirements for good and acceptable practice as enunciated by the regulatory agency to avoid embarrassment and the attendant underhand dealings by unscrupulous and corrupt government staff.

Similarly, you must liaise with relevant professional groups in the area to keep abreast of the activities of your group. They will serve as pillars of support and protection in case of any trouble in your practice.

Good Practice/Integrity and Reputation

Integrity is the quality of being honest and having strong moral principles. It is a prerequisite to a good reputation. Good reputation is very critical in any area of endeavor especially medicine and medical practice, where trust is of critical importance.

Majority of hospital clients are already under stress before coming to the hospital for one reason or the other. Sharing their problems with the practitioners and trusting one for a remedy to their problems are privileges that no one deserves. For attending professionals to engage in shady and unprofessional behavior is tantamount to a gross betrayal of trust. To think that unwholesome behavior will bring quick revenue is a fallacy that will not only sully the image and reputation of the practice and the practitioner but will, in the long run, destroy the practice altogether.

Our experience at MCH is that good practice with goodwill based on an ethical medical reputation attracts good dividends much more than quick, questionable revenues. Not only will a good name and good practice bring patients to your hospital but they will also attract the kinds of experts and professionals who will make your practice a reputable and sought-after place for patient care.

One important way to prevent undue pressure to compromise standards is to avoid unnecessary debts which will introduce all sorts of deadlines or targets for payments. These may bring the temptation to compromise on standards or embark on unwholesome activities. Always remember that a good name is better than silver and gold. Your gifts, expertise and good services will make way for you in the marketplace of life.

Mother and Child Hospital Leadership

The directors and top management of Mother and Child Hospital have tested all the suggestions offered in this chapter in our hospital since inception and we find them practicable and very useful.

Mother and Child Hospital started because of our desire to ameliorate the sufferings of women and children by investing our time, treasure, and talents to provide quality healthcare delivery. We were determined to make a positive impact on healthcare delivery in Nigeria. Our determination, with the grace and mercy of God, enabled us to disengage from the ivory towers to commence a private medical practice in a new environment.

The vision or goals of Mother and Child Hospital is to "Provide high quality comprehensive healthcare services to all classes of people, particularly women and children."

To achieve the vision, we are committed to:

- Ensure high professional standards.
- Make the health of our women and children our priority.
- Provide health care to different classes of people in the community.
- Have the fear of God in all our operations.

This original vision and mission are still our priority, though slightly modified to ensure that all classes of people get quality specialist coverage.

Our aim was to care for the middle-class and some in the upper echelon of society. Therefore, our hospital is located in the middle-class part of Lagos, where we can take advantage of electricity, good road network, water supply, and other infrastructural needs.

MCH was not exempted from financial challenges at various stages of development, particularly at the inception of the hospital. Through prayers and consultations with our partners, we were able to forge partnerships with friendly and understanding investors who believed in our vision and were willing to finance it. The partners have not only contributed financially but they have been pillars of support in every facet of the development of the project. Things may not be like this for everybody but ours has turned out very well. To the glory of God, this hospital is not indebted to any financial institution.

Though integrity is a scarce commodity in our national life today, we have managed to keep ourselves and practice essentially out of corruption and indiscipline by adhering to our vision and mission statements. From inception, we impressed it on all staff not to engage in anything that will contravene the principles of good medical and professional practice. We are law abiding citizens who believe that a good name is better than riches. Good reputation has contributed immensely to patronage by our clients and also helped to attract quality staff and assistance.

Mother and Child Hospital believes that our greatest assets are our staff. Hence, we invest a lot in staff development and training. The management ensures that our staff not only buy into the vision of the hospital, but many of them are also shareholders in MCH. Healthy and happy workforce produces happy and prosperous practice. Ours is like a family environment where we strive to care for each other and our clients.

Mother and Child Hospital is actively involved in activities organized by governments and other stakeholders in the health sector. Our staff are encouraged, supported, and sponsored to participate in activities involving their professional bodies and training to enable them keep abreast with new developments. We believe that informed workers provide quality professional services that add value to our practice.

Mother and Child Hospital management believes that there is no success without good successors. The management is always investing in training and raising competent successors who will take the business to higher level in future.

We have been very blessed and greatly helped by following the points discussed. We hope it can help you too.

There is no doubt that “the finger of God” has been at work in ensuring the success of Mother and Child Hospital (9).

The "God Factor" in Mother and Child Hospital

Of utmost importance in our practice is the place of God – the "God factor." We believe that God rules in the affairs of men and that unless the Lord builds, the builders build in vain. Irrespective of the good efforts we make as mortals, only God gives the increase and overall success. The invisible but ever-powerful hands of the Almighty have produced the tangible results seen in our facility and practice today.

A career in medicine and particularly running a private medical practice can be very rewarding and satisfying because you can make a difference in people's lives. It is also a respected profession and has made the world a better place. At Mother and Child Hospital, we not only alleviate pain and suffering but also put smiles on the faces of individuals and families.

Illustrations of Mother and Child Hospital

The following is a visual "mini tour" of Mother and Child Hospital.

There are four photographs that attempt to briefly show the structure, furnishing, and equipment of this hospital. They illustrate the following:

- The externals of the medical facility (Fig. **1**).
- The inpatients (wards) section of the hospital (Figs. **2** and **3**).
- The operating room (Fig. **4**).

This is the part of the hospital that is visible to not only patients and those who intend to enter the hospital but also the public – pedestrians and those who drive past in the cars and other vehicles that ply the road in front of the hospital.

Many types and ranges of obstetric and gynecologic surgeries and procedures are performed in this operating room.

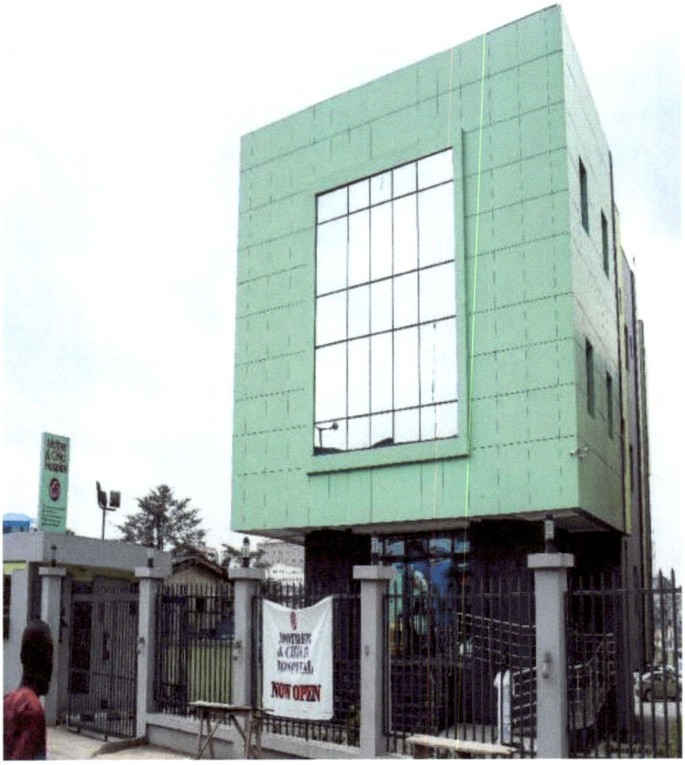

Fig. (1). Front view of Mother and Child Hospital, Lagos.

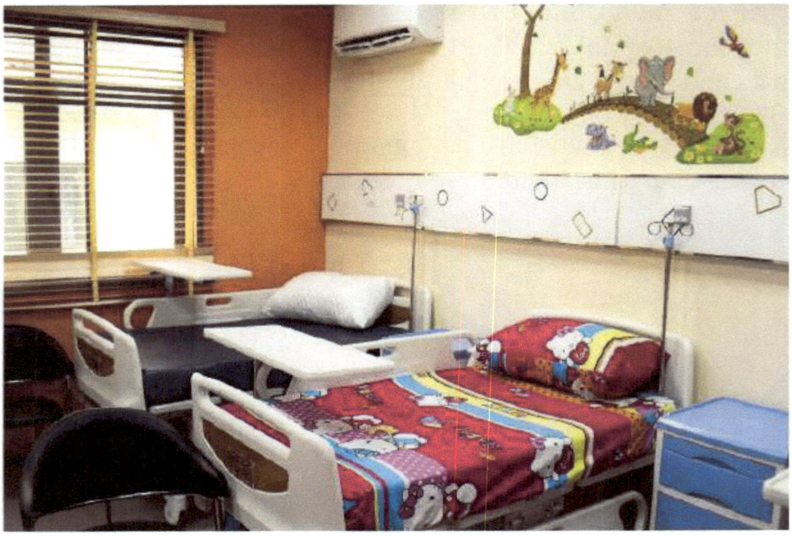

Fig. (2). Pediatrics ward of Mother and Child Hospital

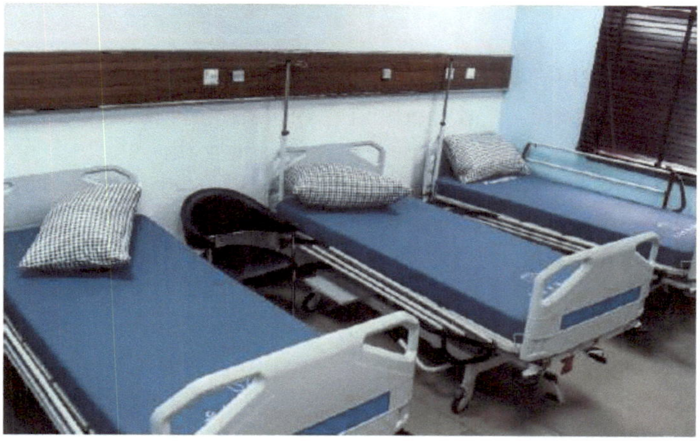

Fig. (3). The Gynecology ward of this private hospital

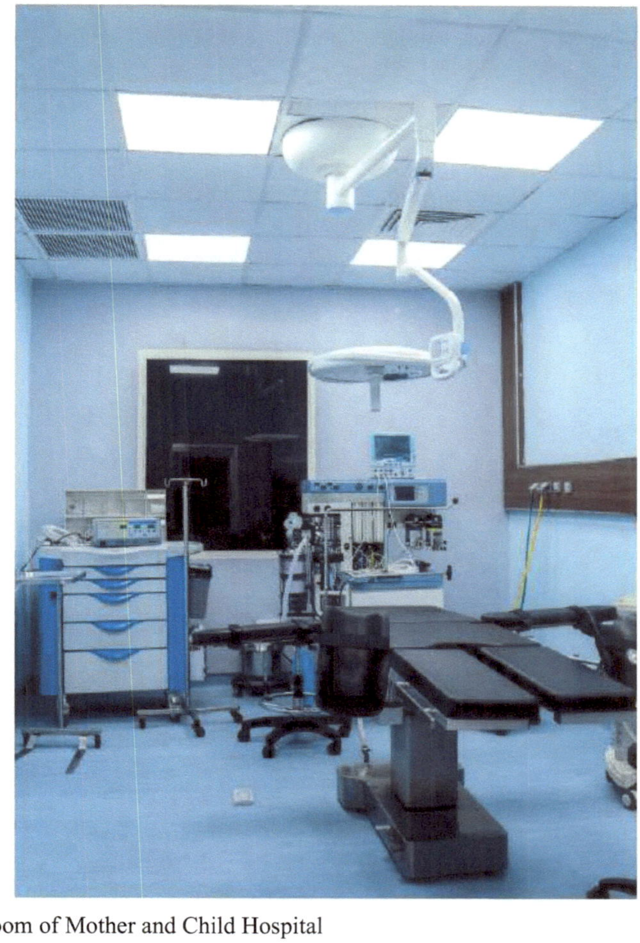

Fig. (4). Operating room of Mother and Child Hospital

CONCLUSION

Success in private medical practice is not an accident. Since it is not an accident, it is imperative for investors and medical professionals to work as a team towards achieving the goal of success. Every private hospital should predetermine its indicators of success and tread the path that will enable them to actualize that goal. Mother and Child Hospital has proved that it is not beneficial to use another hospital as a yardstick but to follow one's own path and stay on course. The patients of a hospital are the best judges of a hospital's progress or otherwise. Although large external features tend to attract some patients, the investor should know that the quality of services a private hospital renders using well-maintained equipment and well-motivated employees is of greater importance than the physical size of a hospital.

REFERENCES

[1] Scarborough H, Fralick PC. Hospital, Definition, History, Types, Services and Facts. Encyclopedia Britannica Published in Google Search 2024.

[2] Fralick PC, Piercey WD. Hospital. Britannica 2024. Available from: https://www.britannica.com/science/hospital

[3] Premium Times. From the archive: Buhari's First Speech As Nigeria's Military Head of State 1983. Available from: https://www.premiumtimesng.com/features-and-interviews/183847-from-the-archive-buharis-first-speech-as-nigerias-military-head-of-state-in-december-1983.html

[4] Nairaland. Coup Speech Of Major-general Muhammadu Buhari 1984. Available from: https://www.nairaland.com/622847/coup-speech-major-general-muhammadu-buhari

CHAPTER 9

Challenges, Success, and Prospects of a Small Hospital: A Story of Rst Clinics Ltd

Inyang Ukot[1,*]

[1] *RST Clinics Ltd., Federal Housing Estate, Uyo, Akwa Ibom State, Nigeria*

Abstract: "Small hospitals" is an expression that many prospective and current proprietors and operators of hospitals might avoid using. This is understandable in a country where it is believed that the bigger, the better. The author deliberately used this expression to buttress the point that "Small" is not synonymous with the quality, significance, or nature of service that a hospital provides. The purpose of using "Small" is also to encourage doctors and non-physician investors to take seriously the prospect of establishing and operating hospitals that are small in comparison with the usual and commoner expansive hospitals, space-wise. To write this chapter, the author conducted a detailed analysis from a search of hospitals and discovered that even the World Health Organization (WHO) and the various governments in Nigeria acknowledge and advocate "small hospitals." In Nigeria, the government allows "Small hospitals" to be sited in remote areas, rural areas, semi-urban areas, urban areas, state capitals, and even the Federal Capital Territory. This alone shows that there is, indeed, a place for "Small hospitals" in Nigeria – and, by extrapolation, in other developing countries of the world.

Keywords: Clinics, Electricity, Employees, Equipment, Maintenance, Medical examination, Nigeria, Planning, Policies, Power, Pre-employment, Procedures, Roads, RST Clinics Ltd., Small hospitals, Utilities, Water.

INTRODUCTION

Impact Clinics Ltd. is a limited liability company that was established in 2007 with the name RST Clinics Ltd. It assumed its current name from 24 June 2025. Some doctors do not want to go through this detailed process that may require the services of an attorney to sail through the requirements of the Corporate Affairs Commission (CAC) in Nigeria. Search for availability of the name of a hospital (large or small) may undergo "rejections" as the same or a similar name may have been "taken" and used by another medical facility. This is just one hurdle. This

* **Corresponding author Inyang Ukot:** RST Clinics Ltd., Federal Housing Estate, Uyo, Akwa Ibom State, Nigeria; E-mail: inyang.ukot@yahoo.com

Impact Clinics Ltd. has since replaced the former company name RST Clinics Ltd.

introduction includes this seemingly small detail as those who start a hospital may wish to watch the progress of the hospital over some time and then apply for registration of the name. Nigeria is a large country with over 200 million people and with thirty-six states and the Federal Capital Territory. Some of the states in Nigeria are as populous as some countries in Europe. It is at the point of application for registration that it becomes clear that the name is in existence in the same State or another State in Nigeria and the name cannot be used. Sadly, this is true even when the name is not a direct match but very similar to the requested or intended name for registration. In this case, the already known name must be jettisoned and another name may be sought. Depending on where the hospital is located and the clientele, people may raise questions as to the "sudden change in name." The curious people may not only be existing individual or corporate clients but also neighbors.

RST Clinics Ltd. did not want to have the above experience and went through the registration process first. Starting off as a legally recognized entity adds a feather to the cap of a new hospital (especially if it is a "Small" hospital); this is because the hospital can solicit a business relationship with any company (large or small). In the case of RST Clinics Ltd., this new and "small" medical company was "retained" by two banks and, soon after, by a multinational oil company.

There is, therefore, an advantage in doing the right things at the right time and being known for diligence, expertise, and thoroughness. RST Clinics Ltd. has, despite its small size, stood the test of time and hardly any client has had a significant adverse experience with us.

The rest of this Chapter describes the challenges and successes of this unique small hospital.

RST Clinics Ltd. is a limited liability company registered with the Corporate Affairs Commission of Nigeria and its registration number is RC 713510. It was registered in October 2007 and started rendering services effectively on 02 January 2008. One of its objectives is the provision of medical services *via* a small medical facility. This company, however, also provides a variety of medical consultancy services when contracted to do so.

RST Clinics Ltd. is a company that operates a medical facility. Medical facilities go by different names and may be classified according to size, level of care that its employees provide, or ownership. "According to the American Hospital Association (AHA), hospitals are licensed institutions with at least six beds whose primary function is to provide diagnostic and therapeutic patient services for medical conditions; they have an organized physician staff; and they provide continuous nursing services under the supervision of registered nurses. The World

Health Organization (WHO) considers an establishment to be a hospital if it is permanently staffed by at least one physician, can offer inpatient accommodation, and can provide active medical and nursing care." [1] In terms of facility size, RST Clinics Ltd. fits into "Clinic," which belongs to the group that may be described as small hospitals.

Concept of the Medical Facility

There is a concept behind any business. The concept varies from one business to another and it may change over time. With medical facilities, the concept may vary based on the owners of the business, the target clientele, the location of the practice, availability of other hospitals or otherwise in the neighborhood, proximity to hospitals that may be similar in terms of areas of specialization of the practitioners or the major specialty(ies) that the facility is set up to concentrate on in service provision. The concept that gave birth to a hospital not only envisions the initial size of the hospital but also the ultimate size. The concept driving the hospital determines how much funds are injected into the project ab initio and how much funds continue to be allocated to it. The amount of income expected to be generated from the hospital also drives the concept.

Concepts dwell in the mind and how well they are configured and nurtured determines how realizable they become. A concept may remain in the mind; it may be short-lived for many businesses, or it may become a reality. The reality may meet the goals of the original concept just as it may exceed them.

RST Clinics Ltd. was almost a child of circumstance. This company was thought of after a sudden and unexpected loss of employment by its eventual medical director. The physician found an unpredictable contract employment at the University of Uyo Teaching Hospital (UUTH), Uyo, just about six weeks after disengaging from the relatively short spell at the multinational company he used to work for. He knew full well that this new employment was an uncertain job that was subject to loss or renewal even after the very first year. To ensure that there would be no room for regrets a second time and that unused time was adequately occupied engaging in medical practice the way he thought fit, the idea of establishing a clinic arose. What kind of hospital would not only be sensible but also attainable under the then uncertain circumstances compounded by limited financial resources?

Many questions were considered and each required obtaining reasonable answer options even if definite answers were not feasible. Would this be a hospital or a company hosting a hospital? Was this going to be just, or yet, another hospital? Would it make sense to locate this hospital in the state capital, Uyo? Since the physical hospital would most likely be in Uyo as the principal medical personnel was in Uyo at the time, where in Uyo would this facility be? Considering the fact that the directors had never lived in Uyo prior to this sudden, unplanned move by one of them to Uyo – while the other was in another state – was it sensible to go beyond the desire to start a hospital when the directors were totally unknown in this city? The only patients who knew the doctor were employees of the multinational corporation where he used to work, and the company had a string of its small hospitals in addition to preferred private medical providers – so who would rather pay for medical services when they and their families were adequately catered for by the company? Who, then, were the possible clients? How would the facility attract prospective clients? What scope of medical services would be provided at the start and what scope would be covered over time? What other interests should the company embrace? What was a realistic size?

One of the greatest concerns lay with the question "How would the company obtain the required funds? This was because commercial banks in Nigeria as at 2007 not only were fixated on any new company submitting "feasibility studies" document(s) that they adjudged as convincing but were also giving loans to private hospitals at the same interest rate they gave to businesses involved in trading; the latter more readily scaled the hurdles of bank requirements including feasibility study reports than a typical hospital could do. Currently, the situation with interest rates in Nigeria has worsened rather than improved. In a Punch News June 27, 2024, article titled "Hospitals can't survive under 33% bank loan rates – GMD president" regarding the Guild of Medical Directors president's speech, Janet Ogundepo reported as follows: "Kuti further described the business environment in the health sector as volatile, uncertain and ambiguous. 'Just last week, two hospitals in Abuja closed due to unfavourable conditions. The cost of operating medical facilities has skyrocketed, while patients' purchasing power has significantly declined. Health Maintenance Organisations have not adjusted tariffs for over two years and the National Health Insurance Authority has not revised prices in a decade".

Most hospital necessities and consumables are dollar-denominated, with exchange rates increasing by over 300%. These factors have made it nearly impossible for hospitals to deliver the required high-quality services [2].

However, there is good news for hospitals in the private sector in Nigeria as in May 2024, there was a partnership between a Nigerian bank and the US Government. The intention of the partnership is to support small businesses in the health sector; such businesses include clinics, pharmacies, and diagnostic centers for the purpose of construction, renovation, and equipment of the facilities. The article does not indicate the specifics of the loans that the bank, First City

Monument Bank, will give to these businesses [3]. The hope is that this will be implementable and sustainable.

Since employees are paramount in running any business, how would the staff members be sourced? What cadre of various staff would be suitable to start and eventually maintain the hospital? What would be the minimum number of personnel to use to commence operations of the clinic? What was the assurance that the business would make enough money to pay the staff? How would the company ensure staff retention? What if we expended so much of the scarce funds on performing pre-employment medical examinations on the personnel and one or more decided to leave within one year – seeing that the cost was free to them but borne by the new hospital? How would RST Clinics Ltd. management inculcate and maintain discipline among staff? How long would be the duration of an orientation program for the initial and all further employees? Would the management succeed in inculcating a positive work culture that would make RST Clinics Ltd. stand out despite being a totally new entrant? What kind of additional training should staff be exposed to? In view of the physical separation between the two main directors of the company, how would the hospital be managed efficiently? What was the right timing for test running the hospital and commencement of the initial services? When should the hospital be open for services – should the hospital be an outpatient facility or one with admission and operative capability? How would the hospital's management personnel ensure that the principles of safety and security are imbibed by all personnel? How would the hospital be run to ensure that nobody is indispensable for its smooth functioning? These were some of the questions around which the concept of the hospital was built.

The above questions can be grouped under the following sub-headings:

Why: Was this going to be just, or yet, another hospital? Would the hospital be run to ensure that nobody is indispensable to its smooth functioning?

When: What was the right timing for test running the hospital and commencement of the actual initial services? When should the hospital be open for services – should the hospital be an outpatient facility or one with admission and operative capability?

Where: Would it make sense to locate this hospital in Uyo? Since the physical hospital would necessarily be in Uyo, as the principal medical personnel was in Uyo at the time, where in Uyo would this facility be?

Who: Who were the likely clients? What cadre of various staff would be suitable to start and eventually maintain the hospital?

What: Would this be a hospital or a company hosting a hospital? What was the scope of services to start and what scope would be covered over time? What other interests should the company embrace? What would be a realistic physical size? What kind of training should our staff be exposed to?

How: How would the required funds be obtained? Since employees are paramount in running any business, how would they be sourced? What was the assurance that staff would be paid? How would we ensure staff retention? How would discipline be maintained? How would we ensure that the principles of safety and security would be imbibed by all personnel? In view of the physical separation between the two main directors of the company, how would the hospital be managed efficiently?

The "Why"

To the question "Was this going to be just, or yet, another hospital?" the answer was that this hospital was not going to be just, or yet, another hospital. It was not going to be in direct competition with any existing hospital or clinic, for the directors had identified a niche that they were convinced that the new clinic would capture. The hospital was conceived to satisfy the peculiarities and inner desires of the owners of the company and the expectations of a class of prospective clients. The hospital was conceived to render the best service that any medical facility of its size could provide. It would come into existence to make the owners, staff and clients happy and satisfied. It was believed that the facility would be one that would allow the medical director not to lose touch with the high level of medical practice he had been exposed to over the years. Another major reason was to make some positive input into human capital development in its immediate community.

The next question in this category was, "Why should there be this new hospital if it would not be run in such a way that nobody is indispensable to its smooth functioning?" It is common knowledge that many clinics and hospitals virtually cease to exist, deteriorate, or, in plain terms, "die" when the original operators die physically or do not even die but cease to function at their usual capacity by virtue of advancing age or declining health. The answer to this real challenge was to create a system of running this medical facility whereby documentation is key and any qualified personnel who is additionally trained in the way RST Clinics Ltd. operates can "hit the ground running." The system is "open" and simplified such that nobody could become an "institution" without whom nothing moved or worked well.

As at the time of writing this account the medical director is still not essential for the facility to open and be operational.

The "When"

Having addressed the issue of "Why," regarding the establishment of this company, another big area for consideration was the "When." We did not want to just arise and start a hospital. We had to go through the processes. The very first was the choice of name of the hospital. Since we wanted a limited liability company, we had to register the company. Each of the names we submitted to the Corporate Affairs Commission was returned as unavailable. It was at the point of near-frustration that we decided to send the three-letter name "RST," and, surprisingly, it was available. That was how "RST Clinics Ltd." went through the registration process and in about three months, the certificate of incorporation was ready. Four months to the eventual test running of the clinic and two months to obtaining the certificate, most of the major equipment and furniture had been purchased in Lagos and delivered in Uyo. "When" was still a challenge because we could not start anything until we had the "Where" to establish our physical presence.

This account demonstrates that the timing of the commencement of a medical facility, even as small as RST Clinics Ltd., may not be within the control of the planners of the business – and this means that provision must be made for this snag.

The next hurdle was obtaining approval to operate the hospital from Akwa Ibom State Government. At the time we were about to start, we applied to the Ministry of Health for an inspection of the facility to enable us to start rendering services. The response we had almost threw us off balance as it was unanticipated. The response was that we should start operations and the ministry would send a high-powered inspection team to the medical facility within the indicated working hours on any official day of work. This was unexpected as we did not know from whom to ask questions on the process of hospital registration prior to this. In hindsight, it was a good policy as it kept us on our toes with the full knowledge of the fact that starting the business with initial staff and not meeting the requirements for registration could take the young, enthusiastic staff, and the hospital backwards. We received a commendation for our organization, readiness, and level of services and were promptly given official approval to operate the clinic. Having obtained the license from the State Government to operate this medical facility we have ensured over the years to have a current operating license. We have made great efforts to ensure timeliness with our financial commitments to the government at all levels is maintained. We also knew that doing the right things with the right people at the right time would save us the embarrassment of going against the Law or trying to do the unethical thing of cutting corners.

With regards to what the right timing was for test running the hospital and commencement of the initial services, we chose to start on 01 December 2007. We used the entire month to test the rented property, the new equipment, the hospital furniture, and the skeletal staff. By the end of December 2007, we were satisfied that we had got it right, and so we were ready to start rendering medical services from 02 January 2008 with the full complement of employees.

The initial experience helped us to address the question "When the hospital opens for services, should it be an out-patient facility or one with admission and operative capability?" We found that it was only reasonable to start with rendering out-patient services. This initial period was when we had to tread cautiously and do what we knew was safest and best at the time. We have not forgotten the initial experience, as that timing was almost perfect. Over time, we would evolve to what we do now.

For a small medical facility that goes by the name "clinic," dying is easy, sometimes convenient, and neither painful nor incapacitating financially. It could be different for hospitals that are big and started big; with such, demise could be slow and certain but imperceptible to both the operators and their clients – unless their top management personnel put in place systems that provide them credible feedback and they are willing, able, and ready to promptly turn things around; time is of the essence in getting it right or getting it wrong.

The "Where"

Like with most other businesses, location could be crucial. So, a fundamental question that required detailed consideration was, "Would it make sense to locate this hospital in Uyo?" This question was relevant because what we conceived was miniscule in comparison with most of the hospitals in the part of Uyo where we intended to site the hospital. Moreover, in Nigeria, and other developing countries or poor economies, the externals are very important. The size of a hospital is very important to prospective clients, as they generally attribute good services to an imposing physical structure. It could be suicidal to locate a small hospital in the proximity of large medical facilities. Location also determines accessibility (or otherwise) to a medical facility; moreover, it also significantly determines the clientele; this clientele could be individuals, groups, or companies. A medical facility that starts in a relatively inaccessible location will likely have the challenges of reach, patronage, and growth especially when the main physicians are new or unknown in the community. A hospital that has made a name over the years could move to a location on the outskirts of the city because of expansion or because it is where it chooses to be permanently – and the hospital would usually succeed in pulling its existing patients and corporate clients to the new facility or facility-complex; not so for an unknown doctor, group of doctors, or their new, small hospital.

In the case of RST Clinics Ltd., the question of "Where" dogged the proprietors. Since the physical hospital would be in Uyo as the principal medical personnel was in Uyo at the time, "Where in Uyo would this facility be?" To make matters worse, none of the proprietors had ever lived or worked in Uyo and hardly knew the city. So the decision was to use the services of a prominent firm of estate surveyors and valuers that obtained from us the specifications regarding the business, the desired clientele, the amount of rent we were willing to pay, and the importance of security. Even with this company it took a long time to get suitable properties and/or locations. Most of the properties were too big, too expensive, or in unacceptable areas. Finally, and surprisingly, a property just popped up – the company that was about to pay the rent suddenly backed out. This pull-out was to our advantage. That was how we got our initial location. The property and location were suitable, but a lot of renovation needed to be carried out on the property – the rent was paid in August 2007 (with tenancy to start from 01 September 2007); renovation work commenced at the beginning of September but did not finish till the end of November. Sadly, but unavoidably, RST Clinics Ltd. had to sink a borehole to enable us to have clean and running water for our business. Interestingly, the property owner requested reticulation to the top floor of the property, and we obliged. We devoted the whole of December 2007 for "test running", meaning that the rent had run for four months before we commenced business on 02 January 2008. In just eight months, the next rent would be due. We had no regrets as this location was readily accessible and easy to describe to prospective clients – some people simply stopped by to make inquiries.

Siting Efficiency of Long-term Health Care Facilities describes a detailed and scientific application of Data Envelopment Analysis (DEA) for determining the location of big hospitals in Virginia, the USA [4]. There is a chasm in the expectations of the over-100-bed hospitals and a five-bed hospital in Nigeria. The only concurrence is that each of the large hospitals and a small hospital in Uyo, Nigeria, were designed to be a "long-term health care facility."

Multicriteria tour planning for mobile healthcare facilities in a developing country is an article that resulted from research using mobile clinics in Senegal, a developing country in West Africa. Senegal has a population that is just about 10 million and this makes its population about 5% of Nigeria. Even in this country that is less diverse than Nigeria, providing medical services is challenging. The authors documented, "Let us restrict ourselves to the case of one single mobile facility (MF). Moreover, we assume here that medical supply for the considered region is to be delivered exclusively by the MF, without support by fixed hospitals or dispensaries." This assumption was theoretical for the purpose of this research. This example shows that even when using a mobile clinic in the design for rendering medical services to a community, the challenges remain, although they may be different. RST Clinics Ltd. planned to operate a small clinic that could render other services. It, therefore, set out to be physical in a hitherto unfamiliar environment while also carrying out a year-long state-wide mobile medical services within seven years of its existence. This required a lot of planning regarding its physical location and another temporary location for coordinating the mobile medical services for a corporate client as corporate social responsibility (CSR) for the latter. The detailed plan for the physical medical facility and the co-ordination of the mobile medical service was pivotal in not experiencing failure on the part of RST Clinics Ltd. and disappointment for the corporate client [5].

The research captured in the article "An Integrated Approach to Multi-criteria-Based Health Care Facility Location Planning" was aimed at addressing the challenge of preventive health care facility location planning. The concept used in this reported study is interesting, although it is highly technical. Its findings are implementable because they support the non-technical approach of RST Clinics Ltd. seventeen years prior to the writing of this chapter. Even when there are adequate funds to establish a medical facility (irrespective of its physical size), it is imperative to take a critical look at what could (and should) be prevented. It may be as simple as avoiding siting a medical facility at a location that has an obvious anthill; the cost advantage of choosing a cheap site may be obviated by the high cost of inconveniencing new management officials, doctors and other healthcare personnel, patients, and patients' relatives. Small hospitals may have the luxury of relocating as a solution to certain challenges, but they could have been anticipated and avoided or prevented ab initio. Professionals or specialists outside medicine should be consulted, even if it is to confirm the observations or conclusions of the proprietors of a small medical facility. RST Clinics Ltd. did this by carrying out wide consultations. Healthcare facility problems can be prevented by a proper siting of the facility [6].

We always planned to have our own property. This became a reality seven years after paying the first rent. The new "Where" for RST Clinics Ltd. turned out to be a near-perfect purpose-built facility we put up in a serene part of Federal Housing Estate, Uyo, Nigeria, meeting our expectations and our clients' needs.

The "Who"

One of the major questions under this sub-heading was "Who were the possible clients?" To the reader who is a medical practitioner, this may appear to be a funny question, but for us, it was not. It was a very real and practical question because who, indeed, would choose to go to an unknown small hospital run by an unknown medical director who was also unknown to the well-established fellow private medical practitioners? The expected private fee-paying patients did not know this doctor and the hospital; neither did organizations nor companies know them.

The preferences and expectations of patients are so important that a private hospital, particularly a small one, must consider them positively. For an existing medical facility, one way to do this is to ensure an improvement in the efficiency of the services that the clinic has carved out for itself [7, 8]. RST Clinics Ltd. got itself set to do this from the time it opened its doors to patients. We felt that this high level of service would attract the clientele that we envisaged.

To make allowance for a safety net or a buffer to absorb the untoward effects of this anticipated twin challenge of identity and credibility, the original concept of RST Clinics Ltd. included a provision for "Who would co-operatively run the clinical affairs of the hospital?" The forecast was for fellow consultants in the teaching hospital to make use of our facility when it would eventually come into existence. The medical director had planned to be available for only two days a week while four days would be open and available to colleagues. Sundays were initially planned to be work-free days. Not even one colleague accepted the offer/plan even though the facilities, staff, and virtually everything they needed were available. That was how the medical director was forced to jettison the original plan of having free days and became available six days a week, almost from the opening of the hospital doors to patients; the time lacuna that was supposed to be covered by external consultants was invariably filled in-house. Immediate provision could not be made to employ and adequately remunerate other doctors, not even young ones. Worse still, a young clinic could not be trusted into the hands of untested young doctors to whom the medical director had not been previously exposed clinically. Therefore, as unplanned and unwanted as it was, RST Clinics Ltd. remained an outpatient facility operated by principally one consultant for many months. Over time the medical director was able to identify two of his senior registrars who could fill the gap of his absence – usually to visit his family residing in another state during the weekends.

The next issue on "Who" was "What cadre of various staff would be suitable to start and eventually maintain the hospital?" We had to consider the pros and cons of employing appropriate staff in terms of length of experience. This was particularly in respect of the staff that would have direct contact with and impact on, our prospective patients and their dependents. Determining the qualities of the initial employees and the subsequent ones necessitated paying close attention to create a match between their expectations and abilities with the expectations and preferences of patients. The clients we expected were upscale individuals who already had a taste of international standards of medical services or would appreciate such services if offered to them [9 - 11]. We had to match prospective employees' experiences with the ability to appreciate RST Clinic's emphasis on quality of service, accept it, and put it into practice. It was considered that employing experienced (including retired) nurses had the advantage of bringing along their wealth of experience. We also deliberated on the fact that (a) we could not get it wrong in the matter of these core personnel; (b) we had specific reasons for planning to establish this clinic as stated above under the sub-section "Why;" (c) we intended to create a corporate identity despite our small size, and (d) we desired to train every personnel in-house after the initial orientation program at the point of or just before assuming duty. It was clear to us that the core and most versatile employees that would serve the purposes of this new and small medical facility were nursing personnel; we also bore in our minds that they could make or mar the clinic right from the beginning. Based on the above considerations we concluded that it would serve our purposes better if we employed young nurses who just qualified as registered nurses (RN) or as registered nurse-cum-midwife (RN, RM). We held the opinion that young, freshly qualified nurses would be more amenable to learning and would not lean on their experience. They would neither have baggage of experiences that are inimical to private medical practice – in which case they would not battle with the difficulty of unlearning bad practices/behavior prior to learning what we would expect them to learn and practice.

The decision was made to start by employing young nurses, even the ones who had just graduated from schools of nursing. We were confident that we could easily train them on the clinic's emphases before the clinic's doors were open to the anticipated patients; this was an add-on to their exposure during their training.

We also believed that, being young, they would appreciate current trends in global nursing practices. Finally, we were reasonably certain that these would be forward-thinking professionals who would benefit from the good foundation we would ensure they receive during the period of service in our medical facility. We, consequently, made it a policy that we would preferentially hire young, inexperienced nurses and train them to handle a wide range of conditions that we expected to have in our clinic. What we decided for nurses would run generally through most, if not all, cadres of staff. Core qualities of every personnel would be the willingness and ability to learn fast, be adaptable, and not be averse to multi-tasking. Nurses, for example, would be expected to learn and know virtually everything about the clinic *e.g.*, how to handle clinic accounts in-house and at the banks, efficient patients' medical records handling, storage, and retrieval. Others included clinic documents and records keeping, performing occupational health tests, safe drug handling, communication and liaison with government officials on behalf of the clinic, especially in the absence of the medical director or director of administration.

We also knew that other staff would render services to RST Clinics Ltd. but would not be our employees – this brought the issue of third-party service providers. Ab-initio, we did not want to incorporate laboratory or radiological and other services into our scope of activities. We, therefore, planned to have meetings with the owners/management of such external facilities so that we would achieve agreement regarding the services we expected, the timing of results, and bill payment plans. All these would involve the "Who" on the other side and we desired to make sure that we were on the same page to avoid disruption of services to our clients – or making a negative impact on the efficiency of services rendered to our patients.

The "What"

At the point of planning the hospital as a limited liability company, we asked ourselves the question "Would this be a hospital or a company hosting a hospital?" After looking at the options comprehensively, it was decided that it should not be solely a hospital but a company that would incorporate a hospital and medical services as its major prop of services rendered. This has helped us in the sense that our original concept does not need to change and, so far, has had no cause to change.

The next thing we had to address was "What scope of services would the hospital start with and what scope would be covered over time?" The answer to this question was the bedrock on which most other questions and answers stood. It was the answer to this question that would determine the location of the hospital, the size of the hospital, the equipment purchased, the staff strength and attendant wage bill, the drug stock in terms of volume and variety, the working hours, and the cost of facility management. The answer was straight-forward: we would start as an out-patient facility that would open from 0800hrs to 2000hrs initially, thus running two shifts for nursing personnel and the medical director putting in approximately two hours in the mornings and doing the major work (or spending the greater chunk of time) in the afternoons/evenings after his contract employment.

Still on the "What" was "What other interests should the company embrace?" We made ourselves open to rendering any services that had a bearing on medicine, whether handling projects for third parties, getting involved in the training of various personnel on request, releasing our medical director in his personal capacity to be a resource person in health promotion programs or even writing documents as long as they would have something to do with medicine and would improve medical services in the community or the health of the population that we serve or have access to.

So the question "What would be the realistic size?" arose. The answer was simple on the one hand but somewhat complex on the other. On the one hand, and for a start, a partitioned three-bedroom flat with standard-size rooms and adequate sitting room was a realistic size, but on the other hand, would it still be realistic after a couple of years? On the other hand, we discovered that while the large size of a property is important and desirable, efficient use of property of any size and giving adequate and timely maintenance to it were also essential – and occasionally more important than its large size. We planned to remain small in physical size even if we had to assume more responsibilities by providing a wider range of services.

The kind of medical facility we were planning and the type of services we projected that we would render it mandatory that we ask and answer the question, "What kind of training should our staff be exposed to?" We eventually concluded that young personnel would best serve the purpose of providing the services we envisioned. To do this, we planned an orientation program to familiarize the staff with everything that we considered essential to their normal day-to-day activities in the clinic. We would encourage them to ask as many questions and as many times as they deemed expedient – and we would give them a time frame of the first month of their employment to get a good grasp of what to do and what not to do. Every fresh employee would understudy longer-serving personnel by pairing to enable learning on the job for the first week. While on the job alone or with another employee, within the next three weeks, they would be guided and assisted by either a fellow employee or a doctor to gain proficiency, especially with new equipment or the ones they are unfamiliar with. Hands-on work would be encouraged during the orientation and initial period of working.

We encouraged continuous training by providing a good variety of write-ups on policies and procedures; these would make veritable training and update materials from which new doctors, inexperienced nurses and other personnel would obtain correct guidance and information regarding the expectations and requirements of the clinic from them. The well-written, laminated, and filed documents would be open, readily accessible and available for use, re-use, and referencing by all staff.

RST Clinics Ltd. ensures indirect training of external personnel, including doctors. By company policy, every in-house employee has the right and is authorized, to encourage external personnel to go by the contents of the clinic write-ups – to which the latter should be directed, should there be any point of contention on their part.

From time to time, training would take the form of a practical demonstration on how to use certain equipment, whether it is newly acquired or has been in the clinic but unused by the current employee or a set of personnel. The vision of this clinic is that everybody should be carried along, and if an instruction is given to an employee, such a directive should not be totally alien to them; the staff may not be the one to carry out the precise task at hand but must be able to help reasonably well when it is required.

RST Clinics Ltd.'s management went as far as engaging a friendly human resources management specialist to render services gratis to the clinic in the form of spending one day on training the entire workforce of the hospital within the first year of existence of the clinic.

The "How"

Being a project that we did not have adequate time to plan finance-wise, one of the challenges that confronted us was "How would we obtain the funds required for this project?" At that point in time, we considered it unwise to source finance from external sources to float the project. We knew that no bank would be interested in assisting a new medical practice; the feasibility study results and report would not meet the stringent requirements of most banks at the time. We also knew that banks would start making loan deductions and accompanying interest as soon as possible. Experience had made it clear that obtaining funds to start a clinic from friends and other acquaintances frequently left a sour taste; these sources were generally worse than banks because they could create personal feuds as a result of not getting their money or the dividends at the time they would expect. Many people wrongly judge the income of hospitals from the number of patients on the attendance register or treat the business the way they treat trading. Finally, many individuals would not give a doctor, or a group of doctors, a loan to start a hospital based on a reasonable repayment time frame but would rather opt for "partnership."

To avoid spending useful and scarce time sourcing for funds with high prospects of getting discouragement in return, it was decided to use the little funds available and start, but stay within the confines of what we considered our well-thought-out strategy of running the affairs of the clinic. However, doing this meant depleting the little funds we had and could have invested the same to yield predictable income. We believed that the risk of using personal/family funds to start the project was reasonable since there was already a buffer of regular remunerative income at the time. So, while the temporary contract employment-cum-prospective clinic was envisioned to be a win-win combination, it could well turn out to be the opposite. We opted for utilizing this source of funds for starting the clinic; we considered it better to lose private funds for a project that could fail than to go down the dark tunnel of indebtedness to any bank or individual.

The next question on "How" was, "Since staff are paramount in running any business, how would they be sourced?" Information given earlier in this write-up tried to show that the proprietors of this proposed clinic knew very little of Uyo but still stepped out to start the medical outfit. The few new acquaintances in the profession did not seem to believe in the project, and some actually voiced their opinion showing the unreasonableness of our embarking on this venture even after it started. It was, therefore, difficult to get recommendations from them in terms of sourcing key foundation staff. What we had to do at those initial stages was officially pay for and paste hard-copy one-page advertisements at the Uyo Main Post Office. We did not know if this would work, but it did. Incidentally, virtually all the young, just-qualified nurses who applied knew themselves, and they informed and invited one another to the initial interview, which took place in the just-renovated and furnished property that was to host the new medical practice. One of the applicants got the information on the day of the first interview we conducted, applied for employment, was allowed to participate in the test and oral interview, and was one of the nurses employed. Over the next couple of years, we will depend on this method of advertising for employees. We did not have social media services we could rely on at the time.

One lingering challenge was the question, "What was the assurance that staff would be paid – and paid promptly and regularly?" This was a big concern because, having worked for a popular and busy hospital in a high-brow part of Lagos many years earlier, the unwelcome reality as an employee was delayed payment of salaries. We had suffered as a family from this situation and would not want any of our employees to have a similar experience; regular and timely payment of staff salaries was part of the culture we envisioned for our hospital.

The next concern was encapsulated in the question, "How would we ensure staff retention?" We could easily figure out that it would be easier to retain experienced staff, particularly nursing staff. By extrapolation, we presumed that retired nurses who could show interest in working for our hospital would most likely have their retirement homes in Uyo. On the contrary, it was an undeniable fact that just-qualified and young nurses would show more enthusiasm towards work and learning new things, but retaining them in the service of the hospital could prove a real challenge in view of family and professional progression considerations. We felt that while they were available to work, we should equip them adequately with the tenets of international best practices of nursing, keep our promises to pay them the agreed salaries and be fair and firm as employers. This decision and the accompanying course of action would prove useful over the years as a few nurses left RST Clinics Ltd. to obtain an additional qualification and opted to return for reintegration into our medical services. Some of the nurses have emigrated to the United States of America, the United Kingdom, and Australia.

On the list of anticipated challenges was the issue of staff discipline. So we had to ask ourselves the question, "How would discipline be instilled and maintained?" In a hospital setting, the issue of indiscipline could be overlooked, causing discipline to be sacrificed for supposed concentration on rendering service to clients. We knew that going that route would be a veritable slippery ground towards a decay in the well-contrived principles for the successful operation of the clinic. We did not want indiscipline to be our stumbling block and so it was decided that discipline should run from the top down, *i.e.*, starting from the directors of the business and filtering down to all employees. We ensured that there would be openness and predictability. We considered double standards when applying disciplinary measures as unwelcome – if staff "a" flouted a rule, the disciplinary measure should not be different if/when staff "b" made a similar infraction. We would have no sacred cows. We would make it clear, for example, that lateness to work, and especially, to scheduled meetings, would not be condoned. The medical director would make sure that not even he would violate the rule on timeliness for clinic matters. We decided that there would be no time book in our hospital and every member of staff would be left to appreciate the disadvantages of looking irresponsible by acting unfairly to colleagues and management. Expectations from staff and responsibilities of management to employees would be properly spelled out in writing. Policies and procedures would, therefore, be open documents for all members of staff to have access to and read. We would, consequently, make sure that nobody would feign ignorance of the contents of existing documents – and our medical practice made no provision for employing illiterate personnel. English would be the language for communication within the clinic. Only when a patient could not be communicated in English would the doctor or other employee communicate with the patient in one of the local dialects.

Two of the biggest issues that we anticipated and had to address were related: Safety and security. So the question was, "How would we ensure that the principles of safety and security would be imbibed by all personnel?" Safety and security were hitherto not matters to bother about in a typical workplace – and certainly not in a medical facility. Things had changed in the country and so we would have to incorporate safety and security concerns into the way we would render services in our proposed hospital. We would ensure that the training of staff would feature appropriate areas of safety and security – this would take place during the orientation, staff meetings, and on a needs basis.

The last but not least concern was how to achieve a seamless functioning of the two main directors of the clinic. The natural question was, "In view of the physical separation between the two main directors of the company, would the hospital be managed efficiently?" We wanted and would only accept an answer in the affirmative – but how would we achieve this? The only answer we considered viable was communication and effective discussion of important non-clinical hospital matters by phone. It had to be because the two officials resided in different states in Nigeria.

Initial experiences

One of the initial experiences of Impact Clinics Ltd. regarding its original name "RST Clinics Ltd." was a battle with incredulity. The skepticism that the majority of the people who stepped into the clinic either as patients, accompanying relatives, or curious visitors had manifested as a consistent and unrelenting inquiry about the name "RST." "What is the meaning of RST?" It was funny and sometimes frustrating to have the same question being posed by completely different people under totally different circumstances and times. Even some of the applicants for employment asked this question at the point when we asked them if they had any questions for the interview panelists towards the end of their interview sessions. Their concern or confusion was almost constant and was occasionally obvious from the facial expressions of some of the enquirers when our equally consistent answer was given to them, "It is just a name." It became obvious to us that for many people, there is indeed something in a name – and, therefore, the name of any business is important, perhaps as important as the quality of products manufactured or services rendered.

The next experience we had was that being a new business entity that was unknown in Uyo; it was not easy for us to do business with other companies. We had conceived, as mentioned earlier in this write-up, that only the absolutely necessary services would be provided in-house while every other service would be given to third parties to handle on our behalf. The only reason we were able to get a laboratory to render services to us and get paid for the services later was because a doctor they had as a good neighbor introduced the medical director and hospital to them. The experience was not smooth initially because they tended to forget to carry out laboratory tests on the few samples from RST Clinics Ltd. in the initial stages, therefore releasing the results late. With time, this unsavory situation was rectified.

RST Clinics Ltd. shared property with residents who had occupied another floor of the property before our leasing of the ground floor only recently. This turned out to be a bad experience. The property had no water supply, though it was on a very conspicuous road in Uyo. Before commencing business, the clinic management had to sink a borehole to have reliable and good quality water and exhibit control of the same. The owners of the property requested that the entire building be connected to the water and we allowed it. This turned out to be a wrong decision as they virtually controlled the water and we had to play second fiddle to our beneficiary. This experience has been useful to us in making business decisions in the future and sticking to them based on sound principles and not sentiments.

The other experience we had in the initial phase of our business was that our calculation regarding the level of patronage was wrong. This left us with young nurses who had inadequate workload to occupy them and their friendship at school started to turn sour in the new circumstance and environment of the workplace. It appeared the clinic was overstaffed and the personnel were therefore underutilized. Having spent so much time and resources employing and providing them with the initial training, we considered it unwise to relieve some of them of their services. The solution was to counsel them and draw their attention to the document the clinic had on relationships among members of staff. Thus, very early in the life of the clinic, the personnel appreciated the fact that the existing clinic documents were not kept for the sake of keeping them but their contents were for guiding or directing the affairs of the clinic.

The young nurses were transiting from student life in schools of nursing where their training was principally in public hospitals. The hospitals where they trained attended to many patients on a daily basis, including patients with emergency conditions. A new private clinic that envisioned and made provision for only a certain clientele and a limited range of medical services at the beginning posed an enigma to the nurses – this was especially as they had to hold the fort in the absence of the doctor. The doctor had to attend to the demand of the alternative employment in the morning hours. The nurses found themselves in a situation where they had to attend to patients and other clients before the latter were directed to the doctor. One experience that these young nurses carried along with them but had to quickly wean themselves from was accepting patients with emergency conditions. They were forced to accept repeated reminders that the clinic could only have patients for observation and such could only be determined by the doctor and not them. They quickly understood that though we needed patients and obviously income, the clinic could not start biting what it would not or could not chew. The solution was to promptly direct all patients with emergency conditions to older and bigger medical facilities in the neighborhood without bothering to wait for or send them to the doctor.

Yet another apparently contentious policy we held, and still hold, based on security and safety, is access control. This meant that clinic personnel must consciously be aware of every human entry into and egress from our facility. Many people who come to our facility for the first time are sometimes irked by this peculiarity. They ask, "Why is your front door closed; is this place not a public place?" We have significantly solved this problem as most of our patients and non-patient clients have come to accept this modus operandi, as uncommon as the approach is, in our direct work environment. Some of our patients have implemented this policy in their homes.

A further initial experience we had was insistence by our female patients of child-bearing age that we could not set up the facility and render out-patient services only. We had to go back to the "drawing board" and consider both the pros and cons of incorporating this added service so early in our existence. We decided to go for it; for clinic management, it entailed injecting more money into the hospital to purchase more equipment and restructure the available space. This new status paid off. Our employees were happy that we chose this option and it made them busier and exposed them to a wider variety of services.

Challenges Over the Years

The clinic has had to grapple with a couple of challenges over the years. What we would consider as challenges occurred after the first three to four years.

Non-payment of hospital bills was one of the biggest challenges we faced. This challenge came from quarters we least expected – from companies and apparently high net-worth persons. As at the time of writing this (ten to fourteen years after), some of these clients have still not paid their bills – and, perhaps, have no intention to settle them. For a medical facility with a large client base, occasional indebtedness may not pose a challenge, but for a purposely slim facility, it could become a threat to rendering efficient services and ultimately to survival. Employees do not know that payment has not been made for the rigorous services they have rendered. The painstaking medical, nursing, and general services rendered would produce desirable clinical results but not an equally desirable response in the settlement of bills. Staff members want their salaries and perks for extra services to be paid promptly, but the money that should have been ensured may have been directed at procuring consumables required to take care of some patients. From these and other challenges, we learnt to be strict in receiving reasonable admission deposits and settlement of bills which could be paid in stages if need be. Private patients with a good track record are excluded from this scheme of payment of bills. For a bigger private hospital, debt recovery is easier as they may have a unit to attend to; this is not practicable in a small hospital. Such debtors seem to know that hospitals that are similar to ours will not spend precious and scarce time, personnel, or funds to recover debt or institute litigation to achieve the same goal.

Within a few years, we recognized that investing in a rented property by undertaking extensive remodeling to make it fit the needs of our hospital was an error. This was because of a continual increase in rent irrespective of the cost the tenant incurred to add value to the owner's building. In our case, the amount we sank into the property was at least the equivalent of two years rent, yet we continued to pay increased rent until the company of estate surveyors and valuers had to intervene and impress on the owners of the property to give us a respite by pegging the rent on a particular year. This was, indirectly, a good challenge because it pushed us into developing and moving into our purpose-built property seven years after commencing business.

Taxes and levies were (and remain) another challenge. These payments have had to be made to the Federal Government, State Government, and Local Government. Some of the levies are difficult to understand as they seem to have no bearing on the kind or level of business an entity like ours is engaged in. Some of the levies are determined in the offices of government officials, giving the impression that the assessment could be plainly unfair. Some of the agents that the Local Government uses have been so different from year-to-year and they are foisted on a business owner without prior notice of a change, placing the burden of knowing the actual agent on the hospital. This means that we have to send an employee to the Local Government office to inquire if the levy slammed on the clinic is a verity and the agent is the right one. We have maintained the policy of paying money into government coffers. We are glad that we are current with the payment of all confirmed bills in the form of taxes and levies due to the government.

Disengagement of young nurses to undergo training for additional professional qualifications has been a recurring challenge. However, having anticipated it, we decided to view this challenge from a positive perspective – the perspective of adding value to the lives and practice of nursing staff. On completing their chosen courses like midwifery, a number of the nurses chose to return and be reabsorbed into the services of our company. The large turnover of nurses has been cushioned by our original idea of creating and maintaining documents that enable any new employee to fit into the clinic after minimal exposure in the form of an orientation program and training. The documents make it easy for them to read, understand, and put into practice; this is demonstrable in the addenda. Documents also helped this hospital as we did not want a situation where the absence of anybody (including the founding directors) would become a problem to smooth operations.

Another way RST Clinics Ltd. has succeeded in buffering the high nursing staff turnover is that the company keeps contact information on virtually all its employees (previous and current) and since the disengagement of most of them was primarily on noble grounds, the clinic does not have any difficulty in making new members of staff place telephone calls to and tap from the experiences of the earlier personnel when the need arises. This applies mainly when they have issues with adjusting to equipment they had not been used to during nursing training or during work in other hospitals.

Critical Decisions/Actions

We have not had cause to make many critical decisions or take critical actions. We believe this is because we had well-thought-out, implementable ideas and vision for the clinic. For example, we never intended to have a big hospital and so most of the things that characterize large and very busy hospitals have never been on our plate and we still have no intention to add them on. We have not had cause to approach any bank for any facility up till now and may not do so in the near or distant future.

One critical decision we have made is to render the highest quality of care in whatever case we take on. Based on this singular decision, the patients who have been exposed to our practice know and are confident that they are in good hands. They know that when we give an opinion or advice or choose a course of action clinically, such is usually incontrovertible, purely professional, and honest as a bonus. Every decision is also without pecuniary connotations to our benefit but only for the patient's ultimate benefit. It is also because of this critical decision that when we recommend referral of a patient to another facility, the understanding is simply that we do not have the facilities on the ground to handle the case from the beginning or due to the case progression, we cannot continue handling the case.

Another critical decision of this hospital is the refusal to leave our patients and patients' relations in the dark over the truth about the condition as we know it currently or as it will turn out to be in the immediate or distant future. We do this with empathy when the case demands disclosure; however, in most instances, the condition is not critical, but getting the correct information and taking the right steps is critical to the welfare of the patient. A patient who comes into the clinic with severe hypertension will be told from the records that the patient has not played the patient's part, like adherence to the prescribed medications. Some of them may give excuses like "I did not sleep well last night," "I am bereaved and that is why the BP is still high," or "When I checked it last week, it was normal, just like the previous week, so I stopped taking the medicine," and "I do not want my body to get used to too much medicine." The truth about the consequences of their actions or inactions sometimes jolts patients out of the dangers they had been exposing themselves to. Some patients do not like it, but many have come to see the virtue of receiving correct information about their health condition. Some information we give is general, but most of it is targeted information – tailored to fit the patient's clinical challenge and circumstance(s).

A critical decision-cum-action we made within the first year of our existence was to yield to the demand of our female patients of child-bearing age to provide ante-natal (pre-natal) care services and commence 24-hour services with admission facilities, including surgical services. That decision has been very rewarding in the sense that we have surprised patients, their relations, and some professional colleagues we have had to call in to render some of the specialized services – their surprise being how an outwardly small facility can render high-profile services and achieve excellent results in each and every instance. Though women made the demand, beneficiaries have not been limited to women, but have included men and children.

The last example is a critical action we took based on prevailing circumstances that occasioned the decision in the first place. This action was to downsize the staff strength; the accompanying action was to place the clinic in what we may call "a state of hibernation." By mid-2016, we noticed that due to a general dip in the economy, companies were laying off staff, private patients were opting for treatment in the more affordable facilities like government-owned general and teaching hospitals in the same city and those who attended private hospitals had difficulty with paying hitherto affordable bills. These realities prompted us to decide to downsize as doing otherwise would make us flout one of our core principles – prompt and regular payment of salaries of everyone on our payroll. We met with our staff and brought the decision to their notice, documenting the proceedings at the staff meeting as usual. The choice of disengagement was voluntary and the few who stayed back did so with the full understanding that the clinic was going to operate differently until further notice. The condition for which we coined the term "state of hibernation" was that on a needs basis, the clinic would resume full-fledged services, like when our registered private or company patients required hospitalization, the 24-hour service status would be activated immediately.

Design of the Clinic and the Services Rendered

Structurally, the clinic was designed to fit the services that were intended to be provided in it. The clinic has an out-patients section and an in-patients section. The out-patients section is at the front part of the building and it is separated from the in-patients section that is at the back by an intervening courtyard. From the design and structure, patients who need just out-patients services may come many times and for years without being exposed to the in-patients section of the clinic. There are a few general features of the clinic, *viz.*: the windows of the hospital have double-netting making it almost impossible for mosquitoes to enter and disturb our patients; the three sources of power ensure that we provide our in-patients with round-the-clock electricity; our dedicated borehole provides the clinic with water every time – and water is an essential ingredient for providing services in medical facilities smoothly, safely, and successfully; a fully equipped separate laundry unit at the back of the clinic to tend to laundry needs of the clinic and patients; engagement of the services of external maintenance technicians who respond to calls about issues on electrical, plumbing, carpentry, air-conditioning, digital satellite television, medical equipment, power generator – their names, telephone numbers, and technical areas are documented in our telephone book, and their telephone numbers are stored in the clinic mobile telephone. Finally, adequate and reliable security services. Security personnel are provided a dedicated gatehouse that is fitted with full toilet conveniences – they have no cause to step into the clinic unless in uncommon situations when their attention is required.

The out-patients' department consists of the reception, nurses' station and doctor's consulting room. The reception is where patients are received and registered, medical records are created or retrieved, and vital signs are carried out and documented. At the nurses' station, injection is given, minor nursing procedures are carried out, and prescribed drugs are brought out to be given to the patient at the reception before the patient departs. A returning out-patient who needs to take an injection or have a wound dressing needs not to see the doctor on duty unless there is a reason to, as determined by the patient, the patient's relation, or the nurse. The doctor's consulting room is compact and it holds all equipment needed for the assessment of most patients – without the doctor moving out of the consulting room; it also doubles as an examination room-cum-procedure room. No patient of the opposite sex undergoes physical examination or even minor procedures by a doctor without the presence of a chaperone. Most minor procedures can be carried out in the consulting room without a waste of the patient's time or the doctor's time. The three parts of the out-patients' department each have a toilet and wash-hand basin while, in addition, the nurses' station has a shower unit. The design of the clinic is such that if, for any reason, a doctor or any of the staff has cause to use the shower, that can and should be done before returning to continue work or returning home at the end of a day's work, or a work shift.

The in-patient department caters to the needs of patients of all ages and both sexes as long as they require admission for hospitalization, whether it be for non-operative cases or operative cases. RST Clinics Ltd. only offers private ward services. The department basically consists of three wards and an extra room. Each room is en-suite and has two windows. There is a wide circulating area that consists of a corridor in this part of the hospital. Though there are three wards, there are five beds. The three wards are planned for two of them to have two beds each, while the third has one bed. Our observation was that most patients want their relations to stay with them even when we tell them that there is no need for that, especially when most times the worst case scenario in our practice is one nurse attending to a maximum of two patients – and frequently one nurse to one patient. The second bed in a room is for a relation as we do not allow patients' relations to sleep on the room or corridor floor. The room that has one bed is for patients who want space and accept that they do not have need for a relation's presence during hospitalization.

A smaller room was incorporated into the in-patient part of the clinic; this room is for use by a doctor when we have critically ill patients or on any day a major operation is carried out on a patient. This arrangement/provision ensures that such patients receive the best attention and that any untoward development is attended to without having time or distance as limitations.

As already mentioned, each of the three wards and the doctor's call room is en-suite. Each of these rooms has a dual water heating facility – the first being the standard wall-mounted electrical water heater and the second a gas-operated water heating system.

Other facilities provided in each of the wards and doctor's rooms are standard: Refrigerator, split-unit air-conditioner, ceiling fan and dual power standing fan (electricity and battery-powered). Digital satellite television is in all wards but not in the doctor's call room – for the doctor; this is featured in the consulting room.

We have resisted the temptation of providing kitchen service in-house as we see it as a distraction and a likely breach of our original vision of keeping the clinic spotlessly clean and free from rodents. We, therefore, use designated hotels and restaurants to provide meals for patients whose relations cannot bring food for them during the admission period. Patients choose whether they want food from a hotel or from a restaurant – hotel staff delivers the food, or our clinic personnel do the pick-up. The cost of food and its delivery is incorporated into the patient's overall bill; this system has been very efficient and has satisfied all our in-patients who opted for it.

By design, RST Clinics Ltd. operating theater (operating room [OR]) is neither a part of the out-patients' department nor of the in-patients' department. The theater is located at one corner of the front part of the clinic that houses the out-patients' department, with ready accessibility to and from the out-patients and in-patients' departments. Its prospective patients may come from the out-patients' department as emergency cases or through the in-patients' department as cold cases admitted preparatory to undergoing operative intervention. Most patients who use the services of our theater get moved to the wards after operations – the only ones who do not need ward admission are patients who require procedures that are beyond the use of the doctor's consulting room or whose operations are minor surgeries. Though a small hospital, we have done caesarean sections, salpingectomies, hysterectomies, myomectomy, open reduction with internal fixation as well as herniorrhaphy, appendectomy, hydrocelectomy, hemorrhoidectomy, and a wide range of surgeries in our operating room.

The other group of services that RST Clinics Ltd. renders is Occupational Health (OH) Services. The ones we are accredited to carry out for an international oil company and its contractors are offshore fitness medical examination and accompanying certification; tuberculosis testing and certification; audiometry and certification and, finally, alcohol and drug use testing and certification. We have done these on oil company personnel very successfully and given the companies credible and reproducible results for more than 10 years.

RST Clinics Ltd. is registered and also structured and equipped to provide external medical services for any third party. The third-party could be corporate or individual. RST Clinics Ltd is well positioned to provide them with reliable and efficient medical services in any community of their choice. Such external services are detached from our medical facility and we prevent unprofessional practices bordering on conflicts of interest. A corporate client for whom we rendered this type of service required us to carry out free-to-beneficiary mobile out-patients' services that covered an entire state in the South-South geopolitical zone of Nigeria and the project spanned one year. This was a very successful venture and RST Clinics Ltd. rendered standard and useful medical service to over 25,000 (twenty-five thousand) patients during the period. We are able to cover two States at a time and provide a wider scope of services or execute more defined and limited projects to meet the expectations of any client and clients' target beneficiaries. Before the Conclusion of this Chapter, there are ten photographs that give a glimpse of the project that RST Clinics Ltd. executed on behalf of the project owner.

As a company, and not necessarily the medical facility aspect, we are also incorporated to render services that are strictly or typically non-medical. We are available to discuss non-medical services encompassing projects like medical structures, assessment of safety features of public and private buildings, and providing advice based on the findings. We are also available to handle publications on/for medical institutions, non-medical institutions, and even individuals.

Growth and the Future

Current Status

In the nearly seventeen years of our existence at the time of writing this chapter, the medical facility of RST Clinics Ltd. has grown. The growth and success have been principally in the realm of providing excellent medical services to our clients. Even when a few patients died in our facility, the relations in every instance did not fail to thank and sometimes commend us for services rendered in the midst of (and despite) their grief. We find this encouraging as it shows that whether a healthcare facility is small or big, patients and their relations are observant, are able and ready to judge and commend good services and attitude.

We do not intend to grow physically and have never had such plans. We also take pleasure in being a positive influence on doctors, nurses, and other cadres of staff that have been or still are in our employ. Virtually all those who have been in the service of RST Clinics Ltd. are not the same – they only get better. While we may not grow physically, we are glad that we have helped and are still helping workers grow in their various specialties. As they grow, we see RST Clinics Ltd. as a part of their growth.

We adjudge ourselves as having grown in the sense that while we are not a household name in the business, we are no longer the upstart in town. We have made a positive impact directly and indirectly on our immediate community as well as the entire state. The successful external medical service we rendered on behalf of a credible and well-known international company provided us with the platform to be projected to the entire state.

The current status of RST Clinics Ltd. is a good one. We had a vision and have actualized every aspect of the mission we gave ourselves. We have earned a good name professionally and in service delivery. The only unfortunate thing is that we have not achieved good success in making all our patients understand certain aspects of our peculiarity. The major departure from most medical practices that are peculiar to us is that we never intended to make patients stay virtually glued to the medical director who has and has always had other passions. That is why the design of the hospital and the services we offer are based on systems and not persons. RST Clinics Ltd. has won the confidence of many similarly experienced consultants in various fields. The idea has always been to work in liaison with them whether the medical director is physically present or not. Unfortunately, this concept seems to be alien, and perhaps impractical, to many patients who tend to feel and conclude that "if he is not there, we shall not go there because we are not sure of getting good services." Sometimes, it is patients' relations who feel this way. There are instances when the medical director received telephone calls from patients and as soon as they were told that he was not on seat or not physically present in the state the enthusiasm of the prospective patient waned – despite the assurances given that good services would still be provided by other colleagues. They do not seem to give a thought to the fact that even when the medical director is physically in the hospital, there are instances when major things are done and he is not part of the team rendering such services. The medical director and management of the hospital sometimes simply make arrangement and contacts for things to be provided and for excellent services to be rendered.

We believe that RST Clinics Ltd. and its present and prospective patients will grow to the point of patients and patients' relatives believing in the systems existing for smooth operations of services in the medical facility, whether in the presence or absence of the medical director.

Plans for the Future

The plans for the future of RST Clinics Ltd. are uncomplicated. The simplicity is predicated on the fact that we are satisfied with the way we have been and still are. Many people would think otherwise – and that is the unfortunate part for them and for us. The desire and plans we have for the future are, consequently, that we shall not achieve a notoriety deserving "has been," or "once upon a time," or even "in the good old days" remembrance. If by hindsight we or our patients and business associates used any of these expressions about RST Clinics Ltd. facilities or services, then that future would be bleak. Simply put, the major ingredient of our plans for the future is to remain relevant – whether in the same location or another location – and in any and every sphere of the services outlined above or additional ones we may be persuaded to undertake. In summary, we plan to make RST Clinics Ltd. remain a preferred primary, secondary, and tertiary healthcare services provider to our past, present, and future clients.

Addenda

These addenda provide documentation that demonstrates a part of the functions of RST Clinics Ltd. We have other documents that are designed to fit our day-to-day work. The forms that we create are simple and easy for our clients to understand.

We have forms that contain the most relevant information and are bereft of details that would reveal too much personal information about the patient. We have forms like pre-employment medical examination forms, which we use to capture the most salient facts about the patient. Others include antenatal (prenatal) registration forms, basic medical examination forms, charts for documentation of inpatients' monitoring, consent forms for operations and surgical procedures, forms for operation and postoperative documentation, referral letter templates, and prescription sheets.

The contents of these addenda are grouped into four, *viz.*:

- Comments by Doctors, Nurses, and Patients.
- Policies and Procedures.

The Procedures component consists of two parts:

- Procedures (Clinical) and Procedures (Non-clinical).
- Pre-employment Assessment of Nurses (Sample).
- Sample of Information for Patients: Safety at Home.

RST Clinics Ltd. had in mind the structure and practices of the Harley Street clinics group. In "Background to this inspection," Harley Street Clinic is described as "... an independent hospital owned and provided by HCA International Ltd. The location is based in London in the Harley Street area. It consists of a main hospital building located at 35 Weymouth Street and uses areas at six other addresses in the immediate vicinity, all controlled by HCA International Ltd. All these areas are covered under a single CQC registered location." [12] CQC is the Care Quality Commission, the independent regulator of health and adult social care in England.

Harley Street Clinic is a world-acclaimed group of practices that covers pediatric and adult services, outpatients' and inpatients' services, and surgical and intensive care for its global clientele. RST Clinics Ltd. had no intention of, or capacity for, replicating the Harley Street Clinic experience but desired to pick a few of its structural excellence and best practices. The addenda of this chapter is in synch with the 2023 assessments of an arm of this medical practice group; these assessments are a small fraction of the rating of the Harley Street clinics group: "The service had enough staff to care for patients and keep them safe. Staff had training in key skills, understood how to protect patients from abuse, and managed safety well. The service controlled infection risk well. Staff assessed risks to patients, acted on them and kept good care records. They managed medicines well. The service managed safety incidents well and learned lessons from them." [12] The policy and procedure in RST Clinics Ltd. regarding even what would be considered minor issues like giving a patient an injection, taking a patient's blood pressure, cleaning the floors, and our unique in-house security arrangement for ingress and egress of patients, third parties, and patients' visitors mirror copy a portion of the best practices of this globally acclaimed medical practice group.

In its small way, and its practice environment with numerous challenges mentioned in this chapter, RST Clinics Ltd. aimed at meeting a part of the following rating of Harley Street Clinics group: Staff treated patients with exceptional compassion and kindness, respected their privacy and dignity, and took account of their individual needs. People thought that staff went the extra mile and care and support exceeded their expectations. Staff empowered people who used the service to realise their potential. They provided emotional support to patients, families and carers to minimise their distress. They understood patients' personal, cultural and religious needs and made sure this was reflected in how care was delivered. Staff supported patients, families and carers to understand their condition and make decisions about their care and treatment. Consideration of people's needs was consistently embedded in everything staff did. Patients told us they valued their relationships with staff [12].

Among the contents of the addenda in this chapter is a verbatim account of the perception, opinion, assessment, or review of verifiable clients and personnel of this small hospital in Nigeria. They represent similarly minded staff and clients of RST Clinics Ltd. who, at the time of writing this chapter, are still residents in Nigeria or have relocated to certain economically advanced countries. RST Clinics Ltd. management and staff have their various religious persuasions but do not because they are not allowed to, project them onto the clients, while the patients (particularly the inpatients) are allowed to practice the tenets of their religion without doing it so loudly as to be a distraction or nuisance to other inpatients.

RST Clinics Ltd. hopes that in the future, the various arms of the Ministry of Health at the state level in Nigeria would go beyond facilities and equipment inspection for licencing of private clinics and do what is the practice in the UK where the state of medical practice of a clinic, hospital, or even a chain of medical practice group (akin to the Harley Street clinics group) is not taken for granted but assessed and reassessed objectively to know the currency of their practices as recorded, once again verbatim, in "We inspected this hospital as part of our risk-based inspection methodology. This service had not been inspected since 2016 and had undergone some changes in its service provision." [12] This sentence alone indicates that there is inspection; the inspection is based on a clear-cut, dispassionate, and objective methodology with criteria one of which is risk-based.

Comments by Doctors, Nurses, and Patients

This sub-section consists of observations of past or present service providers in RST Clinics Ltd. and patients expressing their impressions following their contact with RST Clinics Ltd. Any hospital can receive similar observations and comments from clients *via* email. Both positive and negative comments are useful in helping the management and proprietors assess their clinics' performance and make targeted plans for improvement based on objective inputs and reviews.

"By the grace of God, I have worked in more than ten clinics so far in my career as a medical doctor. RST Clinics Ltd. is one of them.

In the area of leadership, Dr. Ukot is one of the finest human beings I have met so far in my career. He leads by example. He is also a perfectionist. As a result, his approach to the health of his patients, as well as the training of his younger colleagues, is paramount in his daily agenda.

In the course of working with my boss, I enjoyed a cordial relationship with him and all his staff. I cannot remember having any conflict with anyone in RST Clinics Ltd. He has disciplined and well-trained staff.

Furthermore, after spending six years on postgraduate training in Akwa Ibom State, my observation was that the RST Clinic was the best clinic in the State. It had almost all the basic equipment one needs to function efficiently. The clinic was very neat and the environment was conducive.

Whenever I reflect on my life, I always draw the conclusion that God used RST Clinic to make me what I am today. Dr. Ukot exposed me to academic, moral, social, and religious training. The landmark experience I received from him while working at RST Clinic has helped me considerably to reposition two major departments I had the privilege of heading in a tertiary health facility in Nigeria.

May God continue to bless my mentor, Dr. Ukot."

Dr. Egwuda Livinus, *FWACP(FM)*

Senior Lecturer, Family Medicine, Benue State University and

Consultant in Family Medicine and former HOD Family Medicine,

Benue State University Teaching Hospital (BSUTH), Makurdi, Nigeria.

Formerly, SOFPON* Chairman, Makurdi Zone.

Coordinator NHIS**, BSUTH, Makurdi, Nigeria.

Formerly, HOD Accident and Emergency (BSUTH, Makurdi).

*SOFPON is Society of Family Physicians of Nigeria.

**NHIS is National Health Insurance Scheme.

"'Very clean and neat' was my first impression as I was led by a nurse to the medical director's office for my interview. (I had applied for a job as a medical officer). The smartly dressed and friendly nurses also caught my attention. I soon found that RST Clinic was a small but well-managed five-bedded clinic. Looking back at that interview, I'm pleased the M.D. took a chance on me, a post-NYSC doctor, to work in and run the clinic.

The clinic nurses were very polite to patients and other staff and carried out their duties effectively. There was adherence to medical best practices in the care of all patients. Drugs were meticulously selected based on their reputation for efficacy, medical equipment was in good working condition, and medical consumables of high standards were employed. The clinic also invited consultants in various medical specialties to offer their expertise in the care of patients. The patients benefited and recovered faster. The clinic also tended to the healthy by way of very thorough physical examinations and investigations for medical fitness.

There was constant power and water supply, water heating, and catering services for the comfort of the patients. Thus, even without a caregiver or relative, the patient was comfortable throughout his stay in the clinic.

The clinic, however, lacked an in-house laboratory, which I believed would have made patient care even more convenient. The generator was also a source of noise. All the same, it was a rewarding experience."

Dr. Esther N. Ekwo

Senior Registrar in Histopathology,

University of Uyo Teaching Hospital,

Uyo, Akwa Ibom State, Nigeria.

Former employee of RST Clinics Ltd.

"I began to work with RST Clinics under Dr. Ukot, Inyang, in 2008, shortly after my graduation from nursing school. Working at RST really gave me the opportunity to put what I had learned at school into practice and come into contact with people from all walks of life who desired better health. I am truly grateful that he allowed me to be the nurse and caregiver that I am privileged to be today. I definitely owe part of my professional success to Dr. Ukot, Inyang and RST Clinics. During my years of work at RST Clinics, I was truly blessed to have worked under the supervision of Dr. Ukot, who was not just a good medical director but also an inspiring boss. He has remained a role model for not just me but for many others who have worked with him. I am also blessed to have met my beloved husband, who was a patient during my working period in RST and so it has been nothing short of blessings both professionally and socially."

Mrs. Victoria Udemeobong Udosen

Former RST Nurse

"My impression of RST Clinic is that of an institution living up to its expectations and even beyond. My first visit to the clinic was about eight years ago. I had been badly managed by a matron in another clinic, which finally resulted in my medical sojourn to India. There, I met medical personnel who were very much concerned with my recovery, but I could not stay for a long time and traveled home to continue my treatment.

It was in the course of that experience that somebody introduced me to RST Clinic. My first encounter with Dr. Ukot left me with some questions as to whether he was not trained in Nigeria, as I was not in doubt as to his origin as an Ibeno indigene – an Akwaibomite. He and his staff displayed such a courteous and friendly disposition despite my health challenges.

When he prescribed drugs for me, the drugs were dispensed with the entire packets and leaflets in place. I also recall how Dr. Ukot helped me overcome frequent nasal congestion and what was usually referred to as "Change of weather."

Through me, two other people were referred to RST Clinics. They were very satisfied with the place. One of them even married a nurse from there. It is rather unfortunate that Dr. Ukot cannot continue to be present at all times here in Uyo. I hope that one day it will be possible for him to come back."

Ebong S. Udoh

RST Clinics Ltd. patient

"When my husband and I found out I was pregnant in 2010, we began a search for a suitable medical provider. After a few unconvincing visits, we finally drove into the premises of a small clinic on Brooks Street, Uyo, Akwa Ibom State, Nigeria. The environment was clean and the staff extremely courteous and professional, which is rare to find in this part of the country. RST Clinics felt like home with people in white uniforms and stethoscopes. We asked to see the doctor in charge of RST Clinics to ensure we were making the right call and that the doctor was the right person to go on this journey with us.

After 8 years and three beautiful children, all products of RST Clinic's exceptional care, the clinic has maintained the standard we have grown used to. Procedures are followed ALL THE TIME, gloves for every contact and the right quality of medication and equipment for each treatment and feedback is always well received.

Dr. Inyang Ukot, the man behind the wheels, has always been pleasant, willing to educate, and interested in his patient and the person behind the ailment. He is not only a doctor to our family but also a friend and mentor. The story of our medical journey over the last eight years will not be complete without RST Clinics and Dr. Inyang Ukot. Our family is a proud client of RST Clinics and we would like to see RST Clinics grow and duplicate itself. RST Clinics equals professionalism, devotion to the medical profession and passion for human lives."

Thelma and Idorenyin Mbang

RST Clinics Ltd. patients

RST Clinics Ltd. is used in the testimonials to render their authors' contents verbatim.

The rest of the addenda on RST Clinics Ltd. consists of documents that have helped the company in rendering services to our various clients – both patients and non-patients. RST Clinics Ltd.'s functionality and efficient service delivery rest on two major pillars. The pillars are documentation and communication. The documents that form the clinic's documentation are short but contain comprehensive information in a compact, readily digestible format. Some of the areas that they cover but are not described in this chapter are demonstrated by the following names:

Clinical:

- Surgical packs (instruments, gowns, and drapes)
- Consulting room trolley register
- Operation room register
- Operation room items
- Drugs stock cards book
- Drugs supply log book

- Daily use of drugs
- Employees' treatment register
- Form for operation notes
- Consent form for operations and procedures

Non-clinical:

- Working relations among staff members
- Job descriptions
- Invoice (outpatients')
- Invoice (inpatients')
- Receipt book
- Temporary receipt
- Cash register
- Expenditure register
- Duty roster
- Equipment inventory
- Employees' salary register
- Generator maintenance log book
- Diesel supply log book

The general comment on these documents is that every reader should please see them as what is done in, and applies to, RST Clinics Ltd. We are not by any means suggesting that what we do and what we accept are the best ways to go. What has worked for us may not apply to other practices, but we are certain that they have not failed us. Since they have not failed this entity and practice, there is a possibility that they may serve yet others well – and save them the unnecessary exercise of rediscovering the wheel. The proprietors and operators of similarly small medical practices may opt to modify what we have described above and demonstrate in this portion of the book chapter by adding or subtracting content to meet their own peculiar circumstances.

For some readers, this detail may seem to be otiose, but they are deliberately documented and inserted here to assist individuals and organizations who desire to give assistance to some communities in Nigeria or other developing countries. The detail may enable them to know how far they may need to go to ensure that their investments in providing healthcare facilities, even at the most basic level, are worthwhile. Their efforts, if well implemented, would meet the needs of members of their target communities just as clients' reports or reviews give them satisfaction and encouragement on the direction to follow.

The following are some of the documents we created or modified and put to use in our clinic. At least 75% of all available documents were developed and made ready before the day RST Clinics Ltd. started test-running its facility and services. Preparation of these documents commenced five months before 01 December 2007 when the one-month test running of the clinic started.

Policies and Procedures

Policies are formal statements that outline principles, guidelines, and rules governing the operation and conduct within a healthcare clinic [13].

Procedures are detailed instructions specifying how tasks and activities should be performed within a healthcare clinic operationalizing policies into actionable steps [13].

In the setting of healthcare clinics policies and procedures promote and entrench safety not only for patients but also for the physicians in all specialties and other healthcare practitioners that provide direct and indirect support for rendering care to patients [13].

RST Clinics Ltd. considers policies and procedures the foundation for achieving its objective of rendering safe and efficient services to all its clients. These two props have held the company all through its nearly twenty years in operation and ensured the functionality of the clinic and the entire company. RST Clinics Ltd. policies and procedures were documented months before the clinic started operations. Putting them in place made it possible to familiarize employees with them from the first to the current set of employees. Employees following the policies and procedures have simplified and smoothened RST Clinics Ltd. operations over the years.

Rationale for Policies and Procedures

Ensuring that all generators are in working order: Without power generators, this medical facility is like any health center in any remote part of this country. We cannot render satisfactory, or even reasonable, service without functional generators.

Ensuring that engine oil is always available in the clinic: The clinic may go into extended use of generators in cases of absence of public power supply; operating the generator without sufficient engine oil could lead to knocking off the generator engine.

Ensuring that the main entrance to the clinic and the front door are locked or bolted: This is to control the entry and exit of patients, relations, and visitors.

To be nice or civil to everybody who comes into the clinic, irrespective of age or social status: Without these people, we cannot be in business. From their recommendations, we will have more clients and from their negative remarks, we will lose clients.

Ensuring that the clinic is clean and odor-free: Most of our patients want a clinic environment that is like home. The so-called “Hospital smell” is simply an admission of or evidence of poor care at a hospital or clinic.

Ensuring that the overhead water tanks are full most of the time: This ensures a good pressure-head of water to the showers in the hospital. It also makes the hospital have enough water for a long time until any problem with the borehole or its electrical control is solved without inconveniencing the staff, patients, or visitors.

Ensuring that water flows from our taps every time: Availability and proper use of water result in the cleanliness of the clinic, including flushed toilets.

Ensuring that toilet seats are open and not closed with toilet seat covers: This makes it very easy for staff and users of the toilet to check for the cleanliness of the toilet. It is disrespectful to a toilet user to meet an un-flushed toilet by lifting the toilet seat open.

Ensuring availability of toilet tissue paper and clean towels in toilets: It is part of courtesy to guests (even in our homes) to have adequate toilet paper for cleaning up and to have clean paper towels to wipe the hands dry in the absence of an electric hand dryer. Moreover, users of toilets or wash-hand basins will have no cause to let water from their hands drip on the clinic floor.

Ensuring availability and use of “odorless” insecticides: It is a shame to any hospital if an in-patient acquires malaria from mosquito bites before leaving the ward of the hospital;

Ensuring correct entry of patients’ personal information/details in case notes, especially during registration: You earn the respect of the new client/patient and relatives. You have everything to gain by giving the patient paper to print your name and address for you instead of misspelling them. Some patients would opt to fill in the information for you (this is if physical/printed records are in use).

Ensuring that you speak English among yourselves and also to the patient or patient’s relatives (unless they obviously engage you in conversation in vernacular): It is professional to speak English. Moreover, not all our clients understand or speak vernacular, not even those who bear local names.

Paying government levies/tariffs and other bills for utilities like electricity, satellite TV, water, *etc*., when due: Disruption of these services creates a problem that costs much more than the bill that should have been paid as pre-paid or post-paid. The reputation or image of the clinic could be dented or damaged.

Receiving clearance from an in-patient before calling in a visitor: The patient's security is in employees' (especially nurses') hands. The patient must be protected while under our care. Laxity in this regard can lead to serious security threats to a patient.

Providing every in-patient with a new toothbrush, toothpaste, towel, sponge, and bathing soap: We hold this policy because not all patients come from their homes for admission. Some patients come from their offices, *etc*. Even when patients come from home, they may not know that they will be admitted; even if they know they could be admitted, they may not remember to carry along with them items as basic as these.

Ensuring availability of hot water in water heaters: Most patients on admission (and their relatives) will require hot water for one thing or the other.

Giving receipts as soon as cash, a cheque, or electronic funds transfer is collected is mandatory: The date of payment is important and it cannot be shifted to a future or an earlier date. Moreover, the receipts have numbers serially, one after the other. This practice ensures that money paid three days earlier is not recorded after money collected later, *e.g*., today.

Giving only one receipt and no replacement even when loss of the receipt is alleged: Doing this ensures you avoid being held responsible for financial impropriety, including fraud.

When an invoice or receipt is cancelled the original must be stapled to the carbon copy and reference made to the number on the correct/valid invoice or receipt: This ensures good record keeping. Giving another invoice or receipt is duplication and a potential fraud. For some patients, using a POS machine solves this problem readily, but staff must ensure that the clinic does not run out of printing paper.

Carrying out all procedures, *e.g*., preparing injections for administration to patients in the presence of the patient and, when present, the relatives: You save yourself from various accusations related to wrong procedure or intention. This is apart from the fact that it constitutes best practice.

Opening water, food, or drinks in the presence of the patient. In the same vein, water shall be opened and boiled in the presence of the patient: This is simple and common sense best practice; it protects you from accusation of wrongdoing or even foul play.

Correct use of gloves by clinical and cleaning staff: Gloves are personal protective equipment that protect users from acquiring infections from patients; you protect yourself also [14].

Use of Mackintosh consistently: During procedures like phlebotomy or setting up an intravenous line, it protects the patient's clothes and hospital bedding and reduces cleaning work for both the staff carrying out a procedure and the cleaning staff.

Use of apron in the theater (operating room), during phlebotomy, establishing or discontinuing intravenous lines, certain clinical examinations, and procedures: It protects the employee using it from exposure to a patient's body fluids.

Frequent checks to ensure that a large kidney dish, bowl, or tray on the trolley is stocked well with all the required contents at all times: This saves the doctor's time and enables both the nurse and doctor to work efficiently and prevents irritating movement by the nurse or other assistant back and forth to bring one trolley item or another.

Young doctors or nurses think ahead and ask questions (if unsure) when assisting the doctor: This leads to self-respect for the staff in the presence of a patient and smooth, fast work on the patient.

Taking and documenting vital signs: Vital signs patterns are very crucial in patients' management. Additional checks by the nurse on an in-patient when necessary can give a clue as to improvement or deterioration in the patient's condition. This applies even when continuous monitoring takes place, as it is better to notice an early deviation from the normal pattern than wait to be alerted by the machine when the deviation is significant.

Calling a doctor as soon as there is useful or important information to pass on to the doctor: Delay or forgetfulness in passing on information can be detrimental to a patient or the hospital; the information must be documented and delivered even if it is by telephone or intercom;

Ensuring that autoclaves are in good condition and all surgical instruments, gowns, drapes, *etc.*, are autoclaved as soon as possible after an operation: Nobody can determine when the next patient who needs an operation will present in a medical facility with the capacity to handle operative cases, including emergencies, and so we must be ready at all times; always indicate the date on autoclaved items.

Ensuring that an immediate post-operative patient on the theater table is not left without deploying the side rails: Ignoring this could be criminal if the patient falls off the table.

Director of Administration and Medical Director

Section A: Policies (Samples) [14]

- Every employee shall go through interview, which may be oral, telephone, or written – or a combination.
- Medical examination shall be carried out on every prospective employee before assuming duty. In exceptional cases, it shall be done before the first salary is due.
- Salaries shall be paid not later than the 7th day of the next month; where and when applicable, additional variable income shall be paid not later than two weeks after the regular salary is paid.
- The clinic/company shall not give employees salary advances or loans.
- Employees shall not engage in any financial transaction with one another, including buying and selling or thrift/contributions.
- Nursing, security, and cleaning staff shall wear appropriate approved uniforms while on duty.
- Not writing out or giving a patient receipt immediately after the money is received shall be considered a deliberate act by the employee and management shall treat it as such.
- Unless, in exceptional cases, only nursing or accounting staff on duty shall receive money on behalf of the clinic, payment shall be made into the clinic bank account. Electronic financial transactions are encouraged.
- An unconfirmed employee (during the period of probation) can separate from the clinic/company without notice. The clinic can also terminate the appointment of the employee without notice. In either case, the clinic shall pay the employee for work done on a pro-rata basis as of the day of separation; the employee shall not be bound to pay the clinic or the company.
- Employees shall not ask patients or their relatives for a gift in any form.
- Employees shall report any case of harassment in the workplace in writing to the Director of Administration or Medical Director.
- As far as it is reasonably practicable, employees shall not expose their babies and young children to the medical facility.
- Employees shall not eat in the clinic while on duty at their duty posts. They are free to eat in the designated eating area or kitchenette.

- Disagreements among staff shall be reported immediately to the head nurse or the medical director; this shall be done even by telephone. There shall not be quarrels/altercations/fights among staff while on duty. These shall be offenses requiring the application of disciplinary measures.

- Confidentiality of information on our patients and their treatment shall be strictly upheld. A breach in patients' confidentiality by an employee shall be met with appropriate disciplinary measures by clinic management. In RST Clinics Ltd., protected health information is held with utmost responsibility by employees and other personnel who render services to the company regarding its patients [15].
- All employees shall give assistance to doctors who consult in this clinic in one way or another, who carry out operations, or who are called to review patients. Employees shall assist such doctors to understand and fit into RST Clinics Ltd. policies and procedures without offending them in words or actions. Should any such external service provider require a justification, RST Clinic employees should respectfully provide, for their viewing and reading, the appropriate document.

Director of Administration

Confidentiality of Medical Information [15]

- Medical records (electronic or physical/printed) are private and confidential.
- Medical records entered by doctors, nurses, and other authorized employees shall be full and contemporaneous.
- Medical records or parts thereof shall not be physically or electronically taken out of the clinic.
- Medical records or parts thereof shall not be requested for, other than by the doctor – and for direct patient care. If required for research purposes, the medical director shall give approval following written consent by the patient.
- Every clinic staff (full-time, contract, or part-time/locum) shall sign a document committing to uphold the confidentiality of patients' medical records before the commencement of work and handling of patients' medical records folders.
- A patient's medical records or part thereof shall be transmitted directly to another preferred medical provider only following a patient, documented next-of-kin, or legal designate signing a written consent/release (preferably with a clinic witness' signature).
- Patients' medical records shall be released only after the stipulated fees have been paid in full.

Section 26 (1) of the National Health Act (NHA) imposes the duty of confidentiality on the healthcare sector when it provides that "all information concerning a user, including information relating to his or her health status, treatment or stay in a health establishment is confidential."

The Nigeria Data Protection Act 2023 (NDPA) was passed into law in 2023. In the Nigeria Data Protection Act (2023) there are some specific grounds that are of interest to healthcare organizations like hospitals and regulatory bodies. Healthcare organizations may rely on the Act when they process personal data with the objective of protecting the vital interest of the data subject; this is especially when the individual is incapable of giving consent on legal grounds or due to physical limitations or incapacity [16]. The authors also stated that "It is important to recognise that privacy and confidentiality provisions as contained in other health legislation continue to subsist, including for instance, the National Health Act. These remain in force" [16].

Director of Administration and Medical Director

Procedures (Clinical)

Pre-employment Medical Examination

From the inception of RST Clinics Ltd. prospective employees who have scaled the hurdle of employment interview have been made to undergo pre-employment medical examination. The examination takes the form of history taking, physical examination, which starts with taking vital signs [17], and investigations. The latter is predicated on the findings from history taking, physical examination, and the precise job description of the employee. What is presented below is RST Clinics Ltd.'s basic medical examination form. Any small medical practice can adopt it as a template (with modifications) to meet their specific needs.

Pre-employment medical examinations are important to at least:

- Establish the health status of prospective employees.
- Determine whether the workplace would be suitable for prospective employees in terms of its impact on their health.
- Determine whether prospective employees' current health status would be aggravated by their carrying out the work specified in their job descriptions and, if so, to attend to the health condition or do work (or workplace) adjustments to ensure the employees' productivity.
- Determine if prospective employees' current health status would put them at risk or other employees at risk and guide the employer in making appropriate decisions and actions where indicated.

Briefly, depending on other establishments (especially large and multinational corporations), for some employees who are to be employed into designated positions or will be in specified executive positions, the pre-employment medical examination requirements on these prospective employees usually go beyond the scope of basic medical examination in this form and so the contents of this form must not be applied to the letter [18].

"Pre-employment examinations may result in an increase of rejecting job applicants in six out of seven studies." "Better quality evaluation studies on pre-employment examinations are necessary, including the evaluation of the benefits of risk mitigation, given the effect on health and on the financial situation for those employees who do not pass the pre-employment examination." The same article states in its "Implications for practice" that "There is very low quality evidence that supports the general notion that unfocussed medical examinations do not decrease sick leave, but come at a considerable cost of denying employment to a high proportion of job applicants" [19]. The pre-employment medical examination that RST Clinics Ltd. pays attention to is to identify conditions that may put other employees at risk *e.g.*, screening prospective employees for tuberculosis. For companies that want their employees to undergo preemployment medical examinations in our facility, we have consistently advised them against screening for HIV and for early pregnancy and have not included these tests for the prospective employees.

Creating, filing, and Retrieval of Medical Records [14]

Employees at the reception shall be responsible for the creation, filing, storage, movement, and safety of medical records of patients.

Nursing personnel shall be responsible for the above in the absence of medical records officers.

RST CLINICS LTD.

BASIC MEDICAL EXAMINATION FORM

Name (in capital letters): ______________________________

Surname ____________ ***First name*** ______________ ***Middle name*** __________

Date of Birth ___/___/_____ **Age Next Birthday** _____ **yrs.** **Sex** ________

Height ______ **cm** **Weight** _____ **kg** **BP** ___/___ **mmHg** **Pulse** _____ **b/min**

Physical Examination

BMI ______ **kg/m²** **Nutritional status** ______________________

Skin ______________________________

Head ______________________________

Eyes ______________________________

Ears ______________________________

Nose ______________________________

Mouth/Teeth ______________________________

Throat ______________________________

Neck lymph nodes ______________________________

Thyroid gland ______________________________

Chest palpation ______________________________

Lungs ______________________________

Breasts (Partial exam) (R) ____________________ **(L)** ______________

Heart ______________________________

Epigastrium ______________________________

Liver ______________________ **Spleen** ______________________

Kidneys ______________________________

Suprapubic region ______________________________

Groins (R) ______________________ **(L)** ______________________

Genitalia (Males only) ______________________________

Rectal (If indicated) ______________________________

Upper limbs (R) ____________________ **(L)** ____________________

Lower limbs (R) ____________________ **(L)** ____________________

Back/Spinal column ______________________________

Dorsal column ______________________________

Cerebellum ____

Basal ganglia ____

Deep tendon reflexes ____

Other comments: ____

____

____

____________________ ____________________ ___/___/__

Doctor's Name *Doctor's signature* *Date of Examination*

Keep physical medical records cabinet locked except to remove and return patients' folders. If electronic medical records are used, only personnel directly involved in patients' care shall have access to the appropriate section of the medical records system.

In the case of physical records:

- Ensure that no part of the medical records falls off or out of the folder before filing and returning the folder.
- File and store patients' folders gently and serially according to the registration number; similarly, retrieve folders gently (as with filing) to avoid damage to them or their contents.
- Ensure that date and time are documented for every clinical contact.
- Ensure that the order of documentation of patients' records (in-patients or out-patients) shows recent entries at the front and the oldest entries at the back of folders.
- Ensure that periodically there is grouping of portions of physical medical records like continuation sheets, medication charts, observation charts, or investigation results.

Ensure confidentiality of patients' medical information.

The above apply in lieu of electronic medical records.

Director of Administration

Universal Precautions

The principle behind universal precautions is to treat blood and other body fluids from patients and healthcare providers as potentially infectious material;

In RST Clinics Ltd. this procedure shall be carried out by all workers, our employees or not, who could be anticipated, as a result of carrying out their job functions, to have contact with blood or other potentially infectious material;

In the current scope of services provided by RST Clinics Ltd., potentially infectious materials include:

- Blood
- Semen
- Vaginal secretions
- Amniotic fluid
- Cerebrospinal fluid
- Synovial fluid
- Pleural fluid
- Pericardial fluid
- Peritoneal fluid
- All body fluids visibly contaminated with blood
- All body fluids in situations where it is difficult or impossible to differentiate between body fluids

In the circumstances of RST Clinics Ltd. job classifications that universal precautions apply include those carried out by:

doctors, nurses, nurses' assistants, laboratory scientists, and cleaners

In all the situations listed above the worker should be constantly cautious and carry out assigned duties with utmost effort to prevent exposure that could cause infection from infectious material.

Medical Director

Taking Vital Signs [17]

- Welcome and offer the patient a seat.
- Inform the patient that you are about to carry out essential preliminary health checks – this explanation is particularly important if the patient is a first-timer. For patients who are familiar with our clinic procedure, you may skip the explanation.
- Check and document the temperature. Use the most non-invasive method depending on the patient's dressing (which may make the axillary site awkward and inconveniencing), the patient's conviction or otherwise of the necessity of using the oral route, and the necessity of exactness in a febrile patient.
- Check the pulse manually if an electronic monitor is unavailable for any reason.

Use the radial artery, applying sufficient pressure to palpate the artery and count for 15 seconds or 30 seconds and multiply the value by four or two, respectively, to obtain the count per minute.

- Check the respiratory rate if the patient is manifestly ill; otherwise, some well patients may misinterpret it as staring. Respect the cultural and religious bent of the patient; explain to patients before carrying out even vital signs.
- Advise or encourage the patient to sit still for the next step
- Apply electronic BP monitor cuff to the patient's mid-arm skin (not shirt or blouse), paying attention to:
- Align the artery mark on the cuff with the brachial artery *i.e.*, at the medial (inner) aspect of the arm.
- Ensure that the cuff is applied snugly and without folds.
- Inflate the cuff, notifying the first-time patient that though it may feel tight it would be for a brief period and that they should not make sudden movements.
- Read and record in the patient's folder (or electronic medical records) the blood pressure and pulse rate indicated.
- You may repeat steps when required, but document the readings in the patient's records.
- If there is a significant difference between the blood pressure or pulse values when compared with the last entry (or previous entries), indicate in the patient's records so that the doctor will cross-check using mercury or aneroid sphygmomanometer for BP and manual count for pulse rate respectively during consultation.
- Check height in all first time patients.
- Depending on the age of a pediatric patient, check height after at least three months; or more or less frequently as may be required.
- In all walking patients (adult or pediatric), check height with the patient having removed footwear, standing with soles flat, knees straight with hands on the sides, buttocks and occiput touching the stadiometer, eyes looking straight ahead and not up or down. Then press the horizontal arm of the stadiometer as far onto the patient's scalp as possible before reading and recording the height. If the patient's hair or hair attachment does not allow adequate contact with the scalp, indicate that fact in the patient's records.
- Finally, check the weight without footwear and without additional heavy clothing (*e.g.*, jacket).

Head Nurse and Medical Director

Giving an Injection

- Welcome the patient and offer a seat.
- If a child, direct the guardian on providing primary restraint.

- If a child, allay the child's anxiety and communicate the need for the injection.
- Bring out the paraphernalia for preparing the injection.
- Check the patient's registration records and confirm identity. Look for information on drug allergy and confirm any undocumented allergies by asking verbally; if any/additional, document the information immediately in red.
- Wear fresh, disposable latex gloves in the presence of the patient.
- Swab and break the injection bottle/ampoule in the presence of the patient.
- Open sterile injection syringe and needle in the presence of the patient.
- Screen off the patient in the nurses' station/injection room.
- Direct/instruct the patient (or pediatric patient's parent or guardian) to expose the area for the proposed injection on the patient.
- Swab the area to be injected and allow it to dry; if a child, and the patient out of fright "defends/protects" the swabbed area by touching it, repeat the swabbing.
- Inject as appropriate (intramuscular, intravenous, subcutaneous, or intradermal) – if intravenous, apply tourniquet before swabbing the area and inserting the needle or cannula into the vein; then release the tourniquet, inject the drug, and remove the needle.
- After removing the needle, apply pressure with dry cotton ball +/- spots plaster.
- Observe the patient for an appropriate time depending on the clinical state of the patient, level of ambulation, and the type of injection.
- The patient is now ready to leave the injection room, if an out-patient.
- Inform the patient, guardian, or guide of the known common side-effects of the drug.
- Advise the patient to return (or be brought back) to the clinic if any untoward effect is observed.
- Instruct the patient on duration and frequency of the injection with specific time or range of time to return for the injection.
- If more than one injection was prescribed avoid using the same site, side, or area for multiple injections.
- If more than one injection was prescribed the doctor will have ensured that spacing of injection times should not greatly inconvenience the patient or family members.

Head Nurse and Medical Director

Sharps Handling

Sharps have the potential to injure the healthcare professional, patient, and a third party who may be related to the patient or just be a service provider. Sharps are less likely to be injurious to people outside of the care provider and the recipient of care except in extreme cases of carelessness and violation of safety protocol in a hospital setting. Findings from the review of relevant literature by Kenneth *et al.*

were that “challenges in patient safety culture in the Nigeria Health System occur as a result of limited resources, poor regulation, inadequate training and education, and limited use of technology among other factors” [20]. The strategies that the authors proffered for solving the problems are a strengthening of the capacity of healthcare workers by training and retraining, an enhancement of infection prevention and control measures, and putting in place patient safety protocols and guidelines [20].

Sharps are all objects that, in their design and make, are sharp and can therefore pierce or lacerate skin.

A number of these are used in medical facilities, their number and variety depending on the services rendered by the medical outfit.

In RST Clinics Ltd., sharps include piercing and cutting objects/instruments. Piercing objects include injection needles and surgical needles, complete intravenous catheters, trocars with their cannulas, and broken injection ampoules while cutting instruments are scissors and blades.

From the above list, some sharps are disposable while others are reusable.

This RST Clinics Ltd. procedure refers to disposable sharps:

- Personal protective equipment (PPE) mainly latex gloves, goggles, face masks, and aprons must be worn before starting any work involving the use of sharps.
- No needle shall be re-capped.
- No needle shall be re-used.
- No needle shall be removed from its packaging (without or with syringe) without the intention of immediate use.
- No excess needle(s) shall be opened. Needles shall only be opened on getting to, and in the presence of, the index patient, whether in-patient or out-patient;
- No used needle shall be left unattended to, whether visibly or not visibly stained with blood, blood products, or other body fluids of patients.

- No opened needle shall be left on any surface, whether at floor level, body level, or at a height above the reach of hands.
- This procedure shall also apply to surgical blades and scalpels.
- Disposable sharps shall be dropped into a sharp container immediately after each use.
- All disposable sharps shall be put into the sharps container before packing away other items used for a procedure or dismantling the set-up for any procedure.
- Re-usable sharps shall be handled with normal universal precautions from the commencement of their use for a procedure or surgery to their re-packaging for

autoclaving.

- Any injury by sharps shall be reported to a physician on duty, documented, and given appropriate attention immediately.
- Sealing or permanent closure of a sharps container shall be when contents reach the level indicated for doing so, not below or above the level.

Head Nurse and Medical Director

Management of Clinical Waste

Consider every material from a patient's body to be clinical waste; this is because it is not useful for the care or management of the patient, and it should be disposed of.

From the above definition, clinical waste shall include:

- All body fluids are not required, and therefore not stored, for immediate or later investigations.
- Gauze, cotton wool, and gloves that are soaked, stained, or contaminated with body fluids.
- Gloves are used to examine patients or perform minor procedures even if they are not soaked or contaminated with blood or other body fluids.

Put clinical waste into containers and bags meant for clinical waste.

Do not put clinical waste into the regular waste bins or baskets in the clinic.

Discourage patients and patients' relations from putting clinical waste into regular refuse waste bins or baskets but encourage putting them into designated clinical waste containers.

Put clinical waste into the large, clearly labelled container kept outside the clinic building but within the compound when the small receptacles within the clinic are almost full.

Local government agents shall pick up clinical waste for disposal by incineration at regular intervals.

Considering that not only doctors, nurses, and laboratory scientists may be involved in the handling of clinical waste but other workers who were not trained and so do not have adequate information regarding this form of waste although they work in a medical facility or maybe contractors that render services to a medical facility, it is important to ensure that everybody is trained and retrained in this topic that is on safety. Providing them with personal protective equipment

(PPE) may be a measure that is insufficient to address the risk unless training precedes and follows the provision of such equipment. RST Clinics Ltd. ensured that the risk was managed comprehensively.

Medical Director

The following procedure is on operating room items. The singular purpose is to ensure that the RST Clinics Ltd. operating room has the underlisted items before any operation is carried out. These are the minimum, as other items that are required for operating on the index patient are readily added. When some of the items on this list are not required for the operation, there is no harm as they are simply not used.

Operating Room Items

- Fresh disposable polythene aprons – 4
- Large McIntosh for operation table – 1
- Dry cotton balls in galipot
- Cotton swab in galipot and/or Sterets®
- Spots and/or Strips
- Tourniquet and Injection file (if available)
- Green needles 21G – 10
- Blue needles 23G – 10
- 2ml syringes – 5
- 5ml syringes – 5
- 10ml syringes – 5
- Green cannula 18G – 2
- Pink cannula 20G – 2
- Blue cannula 22G– 2
- Yellow cannula 24G – 2
- Green scalp-vein needle 21G – 2
- Blue scalp-vein needle 23G – 2
- Hydrocortisone 100mg. – 2 bottles
- Oxytocin 10i.u. – 5 ampoules
- Ergometrine 0.2mg – 5 ampoules
- Xylocaine® 2% –1 bottle
- Ketamine – 1 new bottle
- Atropine – 2 bottles
- Ceftriaxone 1g – 1 bottle
- Gentamycin 80mg – 1 ampoule
- Water for injection – 5 bottles
- Metronidazole 500mg – 100ml x1

- Normal saline 1L – 2
- 5% Dextrose-in-saline 1L – 2
- 50% Dextrose 100ml – 1
- Savlon® – small bottle
- Methylated spirit – small bottle
- Strapping – 1
- Pair of scissors – 1
- Green-capped bottles – 1
- Yellow-capped bottles – 1
- White- or red-capped bottles – 1
- Universal sterile bottle – 1
- Swab sticks – 2
- Foley's catheter – sizes 14, 16, 18
- Sterile gloves size 7.5 – 6 and size 8.0 – 6
- Sterile gauze pack – 1
- Sterile cotton balls pack – 1
- Sterile gowns 2-pack
- Sterile large drapes with hole 1-pack
- Sterile large drapes with hole 2-pack
- Sterile instruments pack required
- Sterile square drapes without holes 4-pack
- Chromic catgut 2 sutures
- Chromic catgut 1 sutures
- Chromic catgut 0 sutures
- Chromic catgut 2/0 sutures
- Nylon 2, 1, 0, and 2/0 suture sizes
- Vicryl® 2/0 sutures
- Sterile suction tubing – 1
- Suction machine tested and working
- Formalin – keep in cupboard
- Extra universal bottle and/or small plastic container for histology specimen
- Sharps container
- Fresh Dettol® soap – 1
- Scrub brushes – 2
- Shoe covers – 4 pairs
- Face masks – 1 box
- Caps – 1 box
- Disposable scalpel and/or Surgical blade – 1

Medical Director

RST CLINICS LTD. EMPLOYMENT APPLICATION/INTERVIEW FORM

INSTRUCTIONS: PLEASE FILL FORM IN CAPITAL LETTERS & SUBMIT WITH APPL. LETTER

NAME:

____

SURNAME FIRST NAME MIDDLE NAME

DATE OF BIRTH (dd.mm.yr): ____/____/______ **PHONE NO.:** ___________

RESIDENTIAL ADDRESS: ______________________________

____

EDUCATIONAL QUALIFICATIONS WITH DATES

SCHOOLS ATTENDED FROM TO QUALIFICATION OBTAINED

____

1. ____

2. ____

3. ____

4. ____

PROFESSIONAL QUALIFICATIONS WITH DATES

QUALIFICATIONS OBTAINED DATES ______________________

1. ____

2. ____

3. ____

PREVIOUS EMPLOYMENT

PLACE OF EMPLOYMENT FROM TO LAST POST HELD ______________________________

1. ____

2. ____

LAST EMPLOYMENT

EMPLOYER ADDRESS REASON FOR LEAVING

POSITION APPLIED FOR: ______________________________

WHY DO YOU CONSIDER YOURSELF THE BEST CANDIDATE? (BRIEFLY)

____

REFEREES:

NAMES ADDRESS GSM NUMBER ______________________________

1. ______________________________

2. ______________________________

SIGNATURE ____________________ **DATE**____________________

INTERVIEW PANELISTS' COMMENTS

CANDIDATE'S NAME: ………………………………………………………

POSITION: ………………………………………………………………

JOB DESCRIPTION:

…………………………………………………………………………

…………………………………………………………………………

…………………………………………………………………………

…………………………………………………………………………

…………………………………………………………………………

…………………………………………………………………………

…………………………………………………………………………

…………………………………………………………………………

…………………………………………………………………………

…………………………………………………………………………

SUMMARY OF PERFORMANCE

Main Questions by Panelists/Answers by the Candidate:

1...

....

....

....

....

....

....

....

2...

....

....

....

....

....

....

3...

....

....

....

....

....

....

Recommendation(s) by Panelists:

....

....

....

....

……………………………………………………………………………………

……………………………………………………………………………………

……………………………………………………………………………………

……………………………………………………………………………………

Name:…………………………………… Signature: …………… Date: …../ …../

Name:…………………………………… Signature: …………… Date: …../ …../

Name:…………………………………… Signature: …………… Date: …../ …../

RST CLINICS LTD. CONDITIONS OF SERVICE

Remuneration

a) **Gross salary (Naira): ………………………………………………………..**

……………………………………………………………………………

……………………………………………………………………………

(Stated in words, followed by figures)

b) **Official road journeys outside Uyo: ………………………………...**

c) **Overtime rate (Naira): ………………./hour**

Hours of work

a) **Working hours:**

- **Mondays to Fridays: ………….… to ……………**
- **Saturdays: …………………. to …………………..**
- **Sundays: ………………..… to …..………………**
- **For nursing personnel, the standard shift duty hours shall apply.**

Abridged Agreement

The employee shall abide by the terms of employment summarized above.

The above-stated salary shall be a consolidated monthly income.

The employee shall be under probation for twelve months.

Salary shall not be increased within the period of probation.

Any other mutually agreed benefits shall become operative after the period of probation.

The employer shall pay salary not later than the seventh day of the next month.

Employee's signature and date Employer's signature and date

Procedures (Non-clinical)

Non-clinical procedures in RST Clinics Ltd. are in two broad categories *viz.*: purely HR (or administrative) or non-HR and non-clinical. The first two documents are on HR (or administrative) and they are

- RST Clinics Ltd. Employment Application/Interview Form.
- RST Clinics Ltd. Conditions of Service.

These two have just been described above.

Other forms or documents that are used to operationalize RST Clinics Ltd. policies are discussed after these two.

Procedures (non-HR and non-clinical)

Apart from cleaning, which is described here, the clinic has written procedures for cleaning mirrors, washing hand basins, water cisterns, shower and toilet floors, and dusting furniture.

Cleaning

General floor cleaning

- Use a broom, sweeping brush (or both) to sweep gently to avoid raising dust.
- Ensure that the floor swept with a broom or sweeping brush is not wet.
- Sweep the whole area in sections using tile joint lines, *etc.* as markers.
- Ensure all corners and hidden areas are covered.

- Empty refuse into the refuse basket as frequently as required and not only at the end of sweeping.
- Ensure that the refuse basket is lined on the inside with either paper bag or polythene bag. Keep the refuse basket handy throughout sweeping.
- A minimum of three brooms shall be used for general cleaning.
- With one of the brooms, sweep in the following order:
    - Wards
    - Ward toilet floors if dry
- With the second broom sweep in the following order:
    - Out-patients' department
    - All toilets in this department
- With the third broom/brush, sweep the theater (operating room).
- Tie the bag (or bags) containing swept refuse and put them still tied, into the bigger refuse receptacle provided outside the clinic.
- General floor cleaning shall be done at least once in a day, the first being in the morning before commencement of the day's work.

Ceiling Cleaning

- Ceiling cleaning shall be done once every week.
- When done, it shall be before floor sweeping.
- Use long broom that is provided.
- Do not climb any object to help you reach the ceiling.
- Concentrate on ceiling corners to remove cob webs and kill any spider without dirtying the ceiling or top of the wall. If it is necessary, use insecticide on spiders and insects.
- Do not stand right under the part of ceiling to be cleaned.
- Hold and keep the long broom or brush at about 45° to the wall.
- Pick products of ceiling sweeping as described for floor sweeping.

Mopping of Floors

- Use detergent of mildest scent for mopping. Detergent is stored in transparent, dry empty plastic bottles *e.g.* water bottles that have been labeled as containing detergent – and use the caps/cover for measurement of detergent for use in mopping and scrubbing clinic floor.
- Mopping shall be carried out on the whole clinic floor daily.
- Start mopping only after placing two "Wet floor" signs to alert other clinic staff, patients, and visitors.
- Wear non-slip footwear when mopping.
- Ensure that mop (whether wet or dry) and mopping can are clean before the start of mopping.
- Pour detergent into a cap of the plastic bottle now containing detergent.

- Empty one (01) level capful of the detergent into mopping can.
- Add water to half-fill (or to just below the basket level of mopping cap); this should mix the detergent satisfactorily before use.
- Put the mop inside the mopping can after mixing the detergent with water; and not before.
- Do not add anything to reduce or mask odors during or after mopping.
- Gently squeeze the wet mop cloth on the top basket part of the mopping can, removing as much water as possible.
- Never use your hands to squeeze wet mop even when your hands are gloved.
- Mop the clinic floor in three sections, following the order outlined for sweeping.
- Change the detergent water when dirty. As a general guide, change the water after cleaning a floor size similar to the size of the floor of a standard bedroom.
- Discard dirty mopping water in the mopping can into the drains serving the clinic and not into the WC bowl (toilet bowl) or shower bases (shower pans).
- Wash, rinse, and squeeze the mop head cloth after every mopping exercise.
- Keep the washed and clean mop stick with its attached head cloth upside-down (or flat on a suitable object without touching the floor) for the air-drying.

Scrubbing of Floors

- Floor scrubbing shall be done once every week, preferably on Saturday mornings, and completed before commencement of work for the day.
- Start scrubbing only after placing two "Wet floor" signs to alert other clinic staff, patients, and visitors.
- Wear non-slip footwear when scrubbing.
- Store detergent in labelled dry empty bottles of water; labelled as detergent.
- For scrubbing, pour into the mopping can three times the quantity of detergent used for mopping. This means three full (level, not heaped) caps/covers of the empty plastic bottle of water used to store the detergent or another but similar bottle cap.
- Add water to the mopping can, to mix the detergent well.
- Pour on the floor the minimum amount of detergent water solution that is required for scrubbing, and avoid flooding the floor.
- Use scrubbing brush provided. It must be rigidly attached to a long stick with handle at the opposite end to avoid or minimize your bending when scrubbing.
- Scrub the whole clinic floor in sections in the order outlined for sweeping.
- Add one capful of Dettol® or Savlon® to clean tap water in another mopping can. Mop the scrubbed floor in small sections immediately after scrubbing the section.
- Mop the scrubbed floor section with clean tap water until foaming stops.
- Move on to another small section of adjacent floor only after scrubbing and mopping have been completed for the previous small area.

- Empty the mopping can when water is dirty.
- Refill the mopping can with clean water and Dettol® or Savlon®, and use as required.
- Rinse the scrubbing brush and keep it dry.
- Wash, rinse, and squeeze the mop cloth as instructed above; then keep it flat or upside-down to air-dry.

Director of Administration

Pre-employment Assessment of Nurses (Sample)

RST Clinics Ltd. carries out a robust assessment of prospective employees to ensure their suitability for the work that they would perform if employed. The job description and the position of the employee constitute the basis of such assessments. We obtain an application for the position, scrutinize the credentials and the curriculum that candidates submit, and invite them for an interview. When they present themselves for the interview, they are given RST Employment Form to fill physically. At this point the interview commences informally because we can assess the candidate's handwriting, attention to details, focus or otherwise on the instructions, ability to provide the required information within the space provided on the form. The other thing we assess is spellings, use of punctuations, ability to write without errors when under pressure. We give the candidates selected RST Clincs Ltd. documents to read just before the test; we ensure that some of the questions are extracts from the documents. We want to know if they paid attention to the document(s) and read them well while waiting to be invited for the oral interview. This description of our interview process for employment is to give small hospitals in similar circumstances like RST Clinics Ltd. an example from which they can improve and apply in their practices. The oral interview is unpredictable because it is frequently directed by the candidates, unbeknownst to them. Our process is homegrown and fits our needs. However, there are sources from where guidance may be obtained. "Clevry offers a full suite of assessments for your hiring needs with a best-in-class user and candidate experience. Measure the critical attributes in healthcare roles, such as resilience, caring attitude, culture fit, motivations, numerical and verbal reasoning and attention to detail to identify top candidates and potential red flags." [21]

Day: .... Date: ..../ ...../ .... at ....hrs. Duration: 45 minutes

Instructions: Choose **"T"** for the correct statement or **"F"** for the wrong statement. Circle the chosen letter **"T"** or **"F"** just after each Question, *e.g.*,: 75. Sharps are sources of danger in a clinic or hospital. **(T) F**

In RST Clinics Ltd.:

1. Nurses report directly to the head nurse. **T F**
2. Setting up drips is the primary duty of nurses. **T F**
3. The state of the floor of the clinic reception may indicate to the patient and patient's relation how well the clinic is kept. **T F**
4. Ironing should never be done in the afternoon shift. **T F**
5. Bed sheet soiled by vomitus has body fluid on it. **T F**
6. A Cleaner should take universal precaution when mopping blood-stained floor. **T F**
7. Injection is normally given into the iliacus muscle. **T F**
8. Intra-articular injection is injection into a joint. **T F**
9. 75/55mmHg is normal blood pressure in an 18-year-old female. **T F**
10. Fast, thready pulse is one of the indicators of shock. **T F**
11. The nurse should ignore the needs of the outpatient because she has a patient in the ward. **T F**
12. Blood samples and urine samples may not be put in the same refrigerator. **T F**
13. Confidentiality of a patient's medical information means telling your colleagues a patient's medical problem in confidence. **T F**
14. Latex gloves are personal protective equipment. **T F**
15. Vision testing can be carried out on school children **T F**
16. A quiet room is one of the conditions for doing audiometry. **T F**
17. Off-shore oil workers may do both audiometry and vision testing. **T F**
18. Vision testing or audiometry may not be carried out on taxi drivers. **T F**
19. The generator should normally be allowed to run till 10p.m. or 11p.m. **T F**
20. The cleaner should inform the nurse before leaving the clinic on an errand for the medical director. **T F**
21. The washing machine in the clinic is for washing the clothes of both patients and nurses. **T F**
22. The cleaner reports directly to the medical director. **T F**
23. The nurse gives spinal injection to patients before surgery. **T F**
24. The cleaner is not bound to take instructions from the nurse. **T F**
25. A 3-year-child with a temperature of 40.5°C should have a pulse rate of 110/min. or more. **T F**
26. Forced vital capacity is one parameter in audiometry. **T F**
27. Testing the two eyes at the same time tests binocular vision. **T F**
28. BP is best done on the left arm since it is closest to the heart. **T F**
29. A patient with urinary retention is best given 1.5 liters of normal saline

intravenously. **T F**

30. Vital signs are basic but essential indicators of the state of health. **T F**
31. A patient on the transfer trolley should be moved by one person. **T F**
32. A 60W bulb is better for the inverter than a 20W bulb. **T F**
33. The smoke alarm in the clinic is a security equipment. **T F**
34. The security officer should sit inside the reception area to protect the nursing staff at night. **T F**
35. You can take over from or hand over to a colleague without reading and signing the report book since you trust one another. **T F**
36. A nurse can harass a patient sexually by speech, action, or behavior. **T F**
37. It is acceptable to exchange duty with a nurse without telling the lead nurse. **T F**
38. Clinical and safety meetings are not important if you do your nursing job satisfactorily. **T F**
39. A nurse need not learn how to use a computer effectively. **T F**
40. An autoclaved pack may be used four weeks after autoclaving. **T F**
41. To get busy, the doctor-on-call can "study" patients' case notes if there is no patient to attend to. **T F**
42. A friend may keep you company during your morning shift duty. **T F**
43. In a security emergency, run out of the clinic. **T F**
44. You notice the smell of burning rubber and later you see smoke from the ward. You should declare a security emergency. **T F**
45. A company patient is ready to pay the difference to be able to use the private ward. You should allow them though the company's contract with the clinic says "Don't." **T F**
46. You should ensure that a private fee-paying patient pays cash, does funds transfer, or uses the POS machine before leaving the clinic. **T F**
47. A patient with severe acute asthma arrives as you want to give injection to a private patient. You should excuse yourself and attend to the patient with an emergency condition. **T F**
48. A patient spills water on the floor. You see it. You should wait until the cleaner sees it rather than telling her to come and dry the floor. **T F**
49. Two hours before you are to report for your shift you start shivering and feeling cold. You should lie down and sleep since you are not well. **T F**
50. The medical director says something you do not like. You should tell him off in the presence of patients since you know you are right. **T F**

Medical Director

Sample of Information for Patients: Safety at Home

Minor or serious accidents can, and do, occur at home. This write-up is based on the opinion that accidents do not just happen but are caused, howbeit, inadvertently in some cases. This means that with knowledge and some care, a lot of (if not all) domestic accidents can be prevented. Domestic accidents can lead to bodily injury, incapacity, or death; there may be loss of, or damage to, property. Paying attention to what we already know or adding to the information we already have on the subject can significantly reduce the frequency of occurrence of domestic accidents and the severity of their results.

Locations in the house will be used as reference points in this write-up.

Living-room: The living room of most modern residential houses has several types of projecting windows or sliding windows. These windows have aluminum frames that bear glass. Sometimes the craftsmanship of the finished product is not good enough – this may result in wind closing the windows and sometimes rain passing through joints or the rails; occasionally, the windows may be almost stiff, warranting using force to either push windows open or pull them close (or in the case of sliding windows, sliding to open or close). For this category of windows, an effort should be made to ensure that there are metal protectors in the window space, especially when they are external windows of an upper-floor residence. This would prevent injuries from falling through the window, especially of children trying to apply force to close or open faulty windows during a windstorm or rainstorm – or acting when not fully awake. If the living room (or other rooms) has old-fashioned louvre windows, ensure that the levers for opening and closing the windows are not stiff. Forcefully, closing louvre windows sometimes leads to missing the lever and breaking the louvre with one's hand; this may result in cuts. At other times, the resistance suddenly becomes a "give," and forcefully hitting the louvres in that circumstance may cause multiple breaks of the glass and flying splinters of glass that may injure any part of the body. If the living room has sliding doors, the glass portion of the doors is not only wide but also low-lying; the glass should be labeled, marked, or the glass should be interrupted with aluminum – this enables people, especially guests, to mind the glass. Even children living in houses with sliding doors occasionally mistakenly run onto (or through) unmarked glass doors; the use of this type of doors is discouraged and, if they were already installed in an old house, should be removed and a safe alternative used as the replacement. Sharp-edged or sharp-pointed objects should not be kept or left on any chair so that visitors or unwary persons do not sit on them and get injured. People who have floors with rugs should ensure that they do not pass electric wires or cables underneath rugs (between the rug and hard floor) as they may not be aware of wires that have become weak or exposed as a result of cables being stepped upon and walked on for a long time; fires or electric shock may result. Items on shelves, room dividers, or high cabinets should be arranged such that the ones at the reach of, or just beyond the reach of, young children are locked and the keys are kept away; things that are accessible to children or guests who do not know how they are arranged should be light and not dangerous if they fall when lifted, shifted, pulled, or pushed. Pushing may destroy the item concerned while pulling may lead to the item falling on a child or falling on the floor and injuring a child if the item is fragile. When there is a climbing child in the house, chairs and seats should be arranged so that their backs touch the wall, otherwise, some adventurous children could climb chairs and fall off the back.

Dining room: Children should be discouraged from standing on the dining table (or any other table) as they may do the same in the absence of an adult or the presence of an unwatchful adult. This may lead to a fall from a height. Falls from heights, especially with a resultant head injury, may lead to serious problems in the future. A caregiver at home must be trained to prevent falls of young children from heights and instructed and encouraged to report any such falls promptly so that medical attention is sought for and given to children. If the dining table in a house with small children must be covered with a cloth, the cloth should be stuck to the table unless breakable items and hot liquids are not kept on top of the cloth. Small, adventurous children have been known to pull such unsecured tablecloths, causing accidental bodily injury when items on the tablecloths fall from a table edge. Chest freezers are preferred in homes with young children; they have drawers that can be pulled and pushed, and so are safer than deep freezers. A deep freezer has significant open space that poses a danger. This type of freezer should either have keys to lock it when not in use or be kept in a place where the door to that room is locked; when children are all grown, this precaution need not be maintained. For those who take alcoholic drinks, including herbal preparations, they should ensure that unexhausted contents are within their sight at all times. Young children have been known to drink and slip into unconsciousness. Sharp kitchen knives must not be brought to or left anywhere in the dining room where small children can have access to them. As much as possible, only table knives should be used in the dining room.

Kitchen: The kitchen is one of the most compact places in most modern homes. In many homes, storage of items in the kitchen is on the floor, in cabinets, and on shelves at body level and even above the height of human beings – in some instances, where the hand cannot reach unless a person stands on an object. If you have to stand on something, ensure that you do not lose balance and the object you are standing on will neither slip nor cave in; a fall will lead to preventable injury or injuries. It is advised to own and use a step ladder with the proper maximum weight rating for the heaviest person in the house. Water is both a friend and a foe in the kitchen. While water enables us to wash things quickly and satisfactorily, it should not spill or splash on the floor. Water on tiled floors has caused serious injuries from slips and falls – though the background cause was a neglect of simple safety measures. Sharp objects are frequently found in the kitchen; they could be sharp-edged or sharp-tipped. One way of ensuring that injuries do not occur is to keep sharp objects together in a designated part of the kitchen as much as possible. Another way is to ensure that their handles are in good condition. The third one is that there should be good lighting when searching for or trying to pick them up – and when they are used. When they are used, the user must do so with undivided attention. Sharp objects should be kept in the kitchen when there is no choice; the fewer they are, the better. They should be avoided if there are adventurous children in the home. As much as possible, gas cylinder and gas cooker should be separated by secure piping. The cylinder should have its regulator in the locked position after use for the day and opened the next day. The knob(s) of the cooker or stove must not be turned on unless the particular burner(s) is/are intended to be lit and used immediately; this precautionary measure is to prevent gas leakage and fire or explosion injuries. Making and receiving calls with mobile phones should be avoided in the kitchen. Busy homes should use an intercom system, which may be significantly safer than mobile phones. Pots and frying pans, *etc*., must have their appropriate handles rigidly attached to their bodies. Cookware with long horizontal handles should have the handles kept away from the user's body; this ensures that when working close to the pot or frying pan, the handle is not accidentally pushed – as this could lead to spilling hot contents on the body or feet of the person involved. Avoid setting the flame to go beyond the edges of the bottom of the pot as part of the heat/flame may be transferred to the sides of the pot and eventually to the handles, causing unnoticed excessive heat that could lead to a sudden reflex dropping the cookware with its contents – the result could be spilling of hot/boiling contents and resultant hot liquid burns. Proper storage and disposal of refuse prevents or reduces the menace of rodents, ants, and flies in your house. There are more possibilities or scenarios in the kitchen for preventing injury and illness.

Bedroom: If a standing or table fan is used in the bedroom (or living room, dining room) and a young child is around, the adult(s) must be alert so that the child does not stick fingers through the front cover in which case the fast-moving fan blades may cut the child's finger(s). As much as possible, toddlers should be made to sleep in cots to prevent falls, for falls are more likely from the parents' bed. The alternatives are to put a mattress on the floor and keep the child thereon, or if the floor has a rug, something lighter, like a bed sheet, may be placed on the floor covering. If standing fans, table fans, and electronic items like television sets are used in the bedroom, care must be taken that extension cables do not cross the walking areas. They can cause trips and falls when the occupants, whether adults or children, walk in the night; it is worse when the fall involves an older person. When there is no full fall, a broken fall from trips may lead to partial pulling out of the plug from the socket on the wall or the extension cable unit; if unnoticed and unrectified, over time, this may cause an electrical fire or electric shock from partial contact. Most modern bedrooms are en-suite. The associated wash area may have a bathtub or shower unit. Bathtubs have been known to cause drowning if children cap the outlet and want to bathe with plenty of water. Bathtubs also cause significant injuries and even death when there is a slip with a consequent fall. Shower units are safer if they are made of plastic rather than glass and if care is taken to prevent scalding by carrying out a pre-test/setting of the hot/cold water mixer unit. Though it sounds elementary, do not transfer boiling water from the kitchen to the bathroom using an uncovered pot or any open container, as accidentally bumping into another person could cause significant hot water burns. If it must be done, water should be mixed to the desired temperature before leaving the area of boiling the water and moving it in a bucket to the bathroom. In the bedroom, no smoking while lying down must be observed so as not to sleep off and drop cigarette stumps on bedding or clothes.

Staircase: The staircase and staircase landing should have good lighting both in the daytime and at night. Particularly in the night, poorly lit or dark staircases can create safety concerns for both residents and guests. Staircases must have smooth railings, which should be kept clean to encourage use. Avoid making or receiving telephone calls when ascending or descending staircases – a fall from a missed step can cause injuries, including fractures especially for the elderly. Children should be taught not to run up or down stairs. The last tip, though not the least in importance, is that moveable generators should not be operated on staircase landings. Inhalation of toxic gases, especially carbon monoxide, from them, has caused the death of many people.

Hospitals and clinics provide a variety of materials that contain information that the medical practice considers most suitable for them, particularly regarding the relationship between the patient and the hospital. The reference given is to John Street Surgery and the material has a semblance of frequently asked questions for which responses are provided. One of the questions it addresses is “What happens when you are referred by your GP to see a Consultant/Specialist/Clinician Privately?” and, in response to the question, the answer it provides states “This leaflet describes what you can expect to happen if you ask your GP to refer you to see a Specialist privately. This might be a Consultant Doctor, Surgeon, Private GP, specialist nurse, or allied health professional. This leaflet uses the terms clinician and specialist interchangeably to denote a person or team you are seeing privately." [22]

With regards to our patients, RST Clinics Ltd. provides materials on various topics one of which is Safety at Home, just presented in the concluding paragraphs of this chapter. Depending on a current health challenge in the community, the prevalence of a medical condition, or the outcome of treatment for certain conditions, a private clinic or any other small hospital may choose to provide a physical pamphlet or an electronic version on its website for the benefit of patients.

Community Outreach Project Overview and Photo Gallery

The processes that are involved in being trusted to get the contract and carrying out this type of project are long and detailed. Any hospital that is not set up legally and registered to perform this level of services to a corporate organization that is interested in rendering social services yet avoids any form of damage to their corporate image should not delve into it but stay within the confines of rendering regular medical services.

A standard, comprehensive, and specific proposal is required.

The proposal must contain every bit of detail about what will be involved. Examples are:

- A demonstration that the company understands what the entirety of the project entails.
- Evidence must be provided that academically qualified and professionally currently licenced personnel are engaged for the project – the currency must span the project's duration.
- New and high-quality equipment is used. New vehicles should be used for the transportation of personnel and materials to avoid a breakdown that could be very disruptive and rob a location's residents of the opportunity to benefit on that day.
- Ensuring that medications of high quality and with long expiry dates are purchased and used, and that storage of medications is according to manufacturers' specifications.
- Investigations and their results must be reliable and available within the hours of the day's project.
- Standard medical records keeping.
- Protection of confidentiality of patients' medical information.
- A good working relationship and communication among the team.

- Prompt and efficient communication between the team, the medical director, or the designate regarding any challenges while in transit or at the site.
- Interaction with government officials in charge of health.
- Interaction with security agencies and their personnel.
- Interaction with traditional rulers and youth leaders of the various local government areas.
- Establishing and maintaining a good relationship with the host hospitals that the State government authorize to provide space for the project.
- Top-notch administration to ensure weekly, monthly, quarterly and end-o--project reports to the project owner.

These are not all, as there is a close-out meeting at the end of the project. The company must present itself excellently up to and including this component of the project relationship. Getting it right all the way gives the company the opportunity to earn and get a positive review and recommendation for similar and more complex medical projects.

Fig. (**1**) is representative of the activities of the RST Clinics Ltd. team during a year-long, State-wide mobile outpatients' medical services executed on behalf of a corporate client.

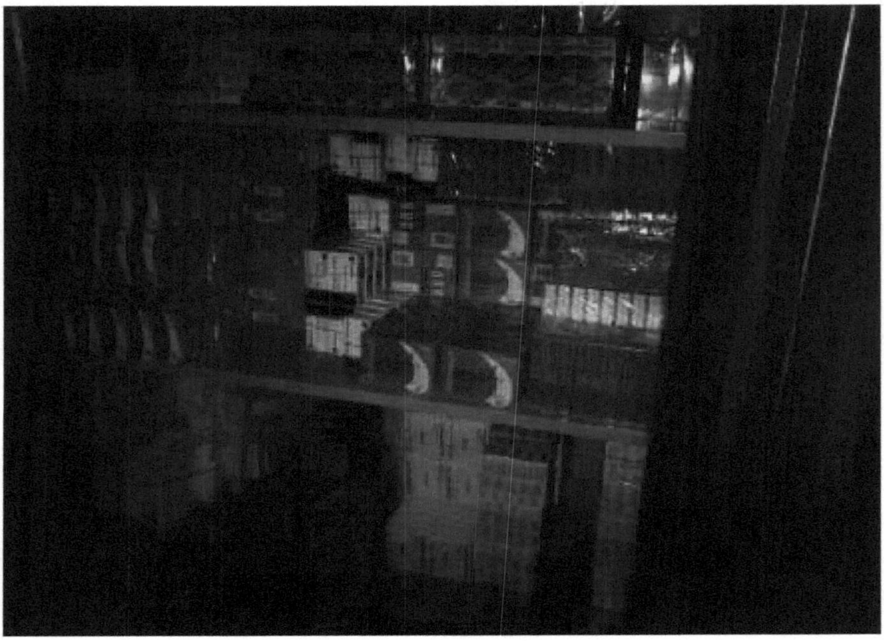

Fig. (1). Storage of some of the project drugs in RST Clinics Ltd. base office.

CONCLUSION

RST Clinics Ltd. has ensured that it started on the right footing as a limited liability company in Nigeria; this makes it a bona fide corporate entity and legal entity.

RST Clinics Ltd. has had its growing pains and made effective use of them.

RST Clinics Ltd. saw the need for creating written policies and procedures even before its registration as a company. This company has benefited immensely from these documents that are made readily accessible to all employees.

By abiding by the laid down rules and regulations at the local government, state government, and federal government levels, this company has surmounted and avoided unnecessary challenges.

This company has proved that following professional principles is a sine qua non to success.

RST Clinics Ltd. has also demonstrated the awareness that what constitutes success is defined not only by an individual or a corporate entity but also by its individual and corporate clients.

Regarding reputation, an established determinant of patients' choice of a hospital, RST Clinics Ltd. would be a new entrant in the competitive private medical practice arena in Uyo, Akwa Ibom State, Nigeria. This new clinic had to establish a good reputation maintain and increase it [23 - 25]. It was essential to provide customized services and part of what was decided that it should offer was home services for a select group of clients [26]; this was not only a high-quality service but also tailored to meet the specific needs of these clients [27, 28]. The variety of outpatient services included well-patients who required occupational health services. The initial location of the hospital was good as it was readily accessible and identifiable even to new clients at night. The clinic has since relocated to its permanent facility in a serene environment that provides it with greater visibility [29, 30].

REFERENCES

[1] CDC National Center for Health Statistics Health, United States Hospital 2024. Available from: https://www.cdc.gov/nchs/hus/sources-definitions/hospital.htm

[2] Ogundepo J. Hospitals can't survive under 33 per cent bank loan rates – GMD president. Punch News 2024. Available from: https://healthwise.punchng.com/hospitals-cant-survive-under-33-percent-bank-loan-rates-gmd-president/

[3] USAID. Press Release. United States Government and First City Monument Bank (FCMB) Enter Partnership to Strengthen Nigeria's Private Health Sector 2024. Available from:

https://www.usaid.gov/nigeria/press-release/may-08-2024-united-states-government-and-first-city-monument-bank-fcmb-enter-partnership-strengthen-nigerias-private-health-sector

[4] Shroff HE, Gulledge TR, Haynes KE, O'Neill MK. Siting efficiency of long-term health care facilities. Socioecon Plann Sci 1998; 32(1): 25-43. [http://dx.doi.org/10.1016/S0038-0121(97)00016-5]

[5] Doerner K, Focke A, Gutjahr WJ. Multicriteria tour planning for mobile healthcare facilities in a developing country. Eur J Oper Res 2007; 179(3): 1078-96. [http://dx.doi.org/10.1016/j.ejor.2005.10.067]

[6] Gu W, Wang B, Wang X. An integrated approach to multi-criteria-based health care facility location planning. In: Cao L, Ed. PAKDD 2011 Workshops, LNAI 7104. 2012; pp. 420-30. [http://dx.doi.org/10.1007/978-3-642-28320-8_36]

[7] Davis BA, Kiesel CK, McFarland J, Collard A, Coston K, Keeton A. Evaluating instruments for quality: testing convergent validity of the consumer emergency care satisfaction scale. J Nurs Care Qual 2005; 20(4): 364-8. [http://dx.doi.org/10.1097/00001786-200510000-00013] [PMID: 16177589]

[8] Torres EJ, Guo KL. Quality improvement techniques to improve patient satisfaction. Int J Health Care Qual Assur 2004; 17(6): 334-8. [http://dx.doi.org/10.1108/09526860410557589] [PMID: 15552388]

[9] Bjørngaard JH, Ruud T, Garratt A, Hatling T. Patients' experiences and clinicians' ratings of the quality of outpatient teams in psychiatric care units in Norway. Psychiatr Serv 2007; 58(8): 1102-7. [http://dx.doi.org/10.1176/ps.2007.58.8.1102] [PMID: 17664522]

[10] Schulmeister L, Quiett K, Mayer K. Quality of life, quality of care, and patient satisfaction: perceptions of patients undergoing outpatient autologous stem cell transplantation. Oncol Nurs Forum 2005; 32(1): 57-67. [http://dx.doi.org/10.1188/05.ONF.57-67] [PMID: 15660144]

[11] Soufi G, Belayachi J, Himmich S, *et al.* Patient satisfaction in an acute medicine department in Morocco. BMC Health Serv Res 2010; 10(1): 149. [http://dx.doi.org/10.1186/1472-6963-10-149] [PMID: 20525170]

[12] The Harley Street Clinic. Independent hospital. Latest Inspection Summary 2023. Available from: https://www.cqc.org.uk/location/1-126955771/inspection-summary

[13] Dune R. What are the policies and procedures for healthcare clinics? Ensuring Excellence: The Vital Role of Policies and Procedures in Healthcare Clinics 2024. Available from: https://www.mandatorytraining.co.uk/blogs/complyplus/what-are-the-policies-procedures-for-healthcare-clinics

[14] 10 important healthcare policies for your facility. Administrative and HR policies. Administrative and HR Policies 2024. Available from: https://www.powerdms.com/policy-learning-center/10-important-healthcare-policies-for-your-facility

[15] Tariq RA, Hackert PB. Patient Confidentiality. National Library of Medicine. National Center for Biotechnology Information 2023. Available from: https://www.ncbi.nlm.nih.gov/books/NBK519540/

[16] Onyemelukwe C, Bhadmus D. Nigeria Data Protection Act 2023: Relevant Provisions for Health Care Delivery in Nigeria 2024. Available from: https://healthlaw.com.ng/wp-content/uploads/2024/03/Nigeria-Data-Protection-Legislation-and-the-Health-Sector-1.pdf

[17] Vital Signs (Body Temperature, Pulse Rate, Respiration Rate, Blood Pressure). Available from: https://www.hopkinsmedicine.org/health/conditions-and-diseases/vital-signs-body-temperature-pulse-rate-respiration-rate-blood-pressure

[18] Fitmed 24. Top 4 Reasons to Conduct Pre-Employment Medical Health Check. Available from: https://fitmed24.com/top-4-reasons-to-conduct-a-pre-employment-medical-health-check/

[19] Schaafsma FG, Mahmud N, Reneman MF, Fassier J, Jungbauer FHW. Pre-employment examinations for preventing injury, disease and sick leave in workers 2016. Available from: https://www.ncbi.nlm.nih.gov/pmc/articles/PMC7163410/ [http://dx.doi.org/10.1002/14651858.CD008881.pub2]

[20] Kenneth KQ, Onuoha US, Dimkpa BM. Patient safety in nigerian health care facilities: A review. In: Asian Journal of Medical Principles and Clinical Practice 2023; 6(2): 224-32. Available from: https://journalajmpcp.com/index.php/AJMPCP/article/view/181

[21] Clevry. Healthcare pre-employment tests. Tests for Healthcare Hiring Available from: https://www.clevry.com/en/platform/assessments/healthcare-pre-employment-tests/

[22] John Street Surgery. Information for Patients attending Private Hospitals and Clinics Available from: https://www.johnstreetsurgery.co.uk/information-for-patients-attending-private-hospitals-and-clinics/

[23] Mohammad Mosadeghrad A. Patient choice of a hospital: implications for health policy and management. Int J Health Care Qual Assur 2014; 27(2): 152-64. [http://dx.doi.org/10.1108/IJHCQA-11-2012-0119] [PMID: 24745140]

[24] Pawlush GG. Health care marketing minicase. J Health Care Mark 1981; 1(4): 49-52. [PubMed]. [Google Scholar]. [PMID: 10254220]

[25] Roh CY, Lee KH, Fottler MD. Determinants of hospital choice of rural hospital patients: the impact of networks, service scopes, and market competition. J Med Syst 2008; 32(4): 343-53. [http://dx.doi.org/10.1007/s10916-008-9139-7] [PMID: 18619098]

[26] Pawlush GG. Health care marketing minicase. J Health Care Mark 1981; 1(4): 49-52. [PubMed]. [Google Scholar]. [PMID: 10254220]

[27] Habtom GK, Ruys P. The choice of a health care provider in Eritrea. Health Policy 2007; 80(1): 202-17. [http://dx.doi.org/10.1016/j.healthpol.2006.02.012] [PMID: 16647156]

[28] Lux MP, Fasching PA, Schrauder M, *et al.* The era of centers: the influence of establishing specialized centers on patients' choice of hospital. Arch Gynecol Obstet 2011; 283(3): 559-68. [http://dx.doi.org/10.1007/s00404-010-1398-0] [PMID: 20180128]

[29] Quintana JM, González N, Bilbao A, *et al.* Predictors of patient satisfaction with hospital health care. BMC Health Serv Res 2006; 6(1): 102. [http://dx.doi.org/10.1186/1472-6963-6-102] [PMID: 16914046]

[30] Campbell JL, Ramsay J, Green J. Age, gender, socioeconomic, and ethnic differences in patients' assessments of primary health care. Qual Health Care 2001; 10(2): 90-5. [http://dx.doi.org/10.1136/qhc.10.2.90] [PMID: 11389317]

SUBJECT INDEX

I

L

M

N

O

P

Q

R

S

T

U

V

W

www.ingramcontent.com/pod-product-compliance
Lightning Source LLC
LaVergne TN
LVHW070949210926
848482LV00002B/152
9798898812065